Why We Revolt

A patient revolution for careful and kind care

Victor Montori

Published by
The Patient Revolution
Rochester, Minnesota, U.S.A.

Paperback edition – October 2017
ISBN: 0999394819
ISBN-13: 978-0999394816 (Patient Revolution, The)

Advanced praise for *Why We Revolt*

We revolt because our health — our very lives — matter.
Why We Revolt does not serve as a blueprint but as an inspiration
for patients and clinicians who are ready to pry open the idea of
"healthcare" and make it about actual health and care. This book
is a necessary catalyst for conversations that will revolutionize
patient care.

> – Kerri Sparling, diabetes patient advocate
>   and creator of sixuntilme.com

This profoundly humanistic examination of what has gone wrong in
medicine has the diagnosis just right. This book is for everyone who
will ever be a patient, for every health professional, and for every
administrator and policy-maker.

> – Gordon Guyatt, physician and researcher,
>   father of evidence-based medicine

I went into medicine to interact with real, unique, emotive humans.
Why We Revolt brings healthcare back to this primary love of and
care for patients.

> – Sara Segner, medical student

Montori begins with a gut punch that stays with you throughout
this powerful, sobering, eye-opening book. After expertly
diagnosing the roots of "industrial healthcare" problems, he
passionately plots a patient revolution. Policy makers, clinicians,
patients, and journalists should set aside the very little time needed
to absorb this gem and learn from its lessons.

> – Gary Schwitzer, journalist and publisher
>   of healthnewsreview.org

If someone gave you this book, they were probably hoping to advance a patient revolution.

I hope you can do the same.

Keep this copy, get another one, and give it to someone else.

To share your stories or send me a note:
victor@patientrevolution.org or @vmontori on Twitter.

To review notes and links to online resources for each chapter:
patientrevolution.org/whywerevolt

To join and contribute to The Patient Revolution:
patientrevolution.org

Thank you, and take care.

V

Contents

To my sons

Introduction – Revolt

Orwell proposed that one must write, among other reasons, to "see things as they are, to find out true facts and store them up for the use of posterity." This book arises from my need to do just that. And what I see is that healthcare has corrupted its mission, it has stopped caring, and I am not going along with it. It is time for a patient revolution to bring about careful and kind patient care for all.

This book also documents my sense of what is wrong about industrial healthcare. Industrial healthcare fails to notice patients. It standardizes practices for *patients like this*, rather than caring for *this patient*. Efficient specialization and narrow job definitions drive industrial healthcare's focus toward organs, diseases, or test results. Rigid protocols and fear of deviating from them miss the person. Systems that prioritize access and volume place very little value on the length and depth of the interaction between patients and clinicians. Forcing encounters to be brief and shallow speeds patients through consultations in which clinicians cannot appreciate their patients' situation clearly. Failure to notice is also the effect of encounters bloated with industrial agendas, such as documentation and billing, which draw attention away from patients and toward the computer monitor, distracting from care to document it.

How does care then take place when the patient is unnoticed, sometimes nothing more than a blur? Judging from the stories that clinicians and patients tell, care happens almost by mistake, when someone takes exception to or ignores protocols. In the absence of these accidents, of these caring mistakes, the industry is capable of harm through unintentional cruelty. As it makes care accidental and cruelty incidental, industrial healthcare marches on to produce fortune and power. By focusing on its industrial goals, healthcare forgoes caring.

The harm is not only to patients. Industrial healthcare is killing the healer's soul. Enforced productivity depletes clinicians. Under efficiency pressures, clinicians cannot draw meaning from fleeting patient visits. They cannot get support from sped-up colleagues. They feel abused and without love — and unable to love. Burnout, divorce, and suicide become inherent to the work of health care, the healer's curse. Industrial healthcare has stopped caring for both patients and clinicians, everyone at the frontline.

Many of my patients, my family, and I have benefited greatly from the wonders of modern healthcare: expert surgical teams, clean and efficient facilities with the necessary equipment, carefully organized services that collaborate and coordinate, well-trained professionals who cordially attend to the sick and invest each one with dignity. All this is possible. It happens, just not routinely or by default. This is the *should be* that I have the great fortune of enjoying on good days.

On bad days, this *should be* lurks between tightly scheduled slots, in the furtive half-smile of another clinician rushing on to their next patient, in the sigh of the staff who had hoped to give more prompt service. It screams from the notes I get from family members or their friends asking for a second opinion or telling their stories, some of them horrific tales of perfect medicine for the wrong person or for the wrong problem. It pulls at my heart when I see what has happened to the patient in front of me: files filled with the results of tests and procedures, 12 medications, multiple specialists, and notes that reveal that no one ever stopped to notice. On many days, I am afraid I am that clinician, that cog of the machine, the one who fails to notice.

Simply noticing and acting on what is noticed makes patients more likely to receive care that makes intellectual, emotional, and practical sense to them — care that responds to their needs and is consistent with their views of the world and their lives. This is care that recognizes and respects that patients may need to devote their scarce time, energy, and attention to matters that compete in priority with the administrative and self-care tasks healthcare has delegated to patients. This is care that responds with competence, science, creativity, and humanity to advance each patient's situation without overwhelming patients or creating new ills.

The words in these chapters, I hope, will ignite in you the urgent need to join us in destroying the difference between *what is* and *what should be*. In abolishing accidental care and incidental cruelty. In making care the intentional end of our work, not the means to achieve industrial goals. In ensuring our best medicine reaches everyone who needs it. Clinicians, anyone honored by the possibility to care, must notice and act toward each person in need of their care. They must appreciate each person's circumstance, concerns, contexts, biology, and biography. To appreciate each patient, the clinician must throw moorings that, for a moment, partner the boats. Traversing rough waters unhurriedly, elegantly, together, patient and clinician can, with compassion and competence, co-create a trajectory for the patient that advances her particular situation. Such careful and kind care for all must be the end result of a patient revolution.

This book is organized as a series of essays. Part One discusses the ills of industrial healthcare, the targets of the revolution: cruelty, blur, burden, and greed. Part Two discusses some antidotes: elegance, solidarity, love, and integrity. The remainder concern careful and timeless care. The book concludes with images of a revolution of conversations and the cathedrals of care that it will build.

This book is not a research report or a lay summary of expert and rigorous observations. This is unusual for me, a clinician who has spent considerable time conducting and publishing research. I am sure that the decade-long work my team and I have conducted directly influences how I notice and document this world. As an academic, I have endeavored to be rigorous and reasonable. But this volume is not dispassionate, impartial, or academic. This is a soulful download, an honest account. In finding the words to articulate what I see, in trying to persuade you to notice, I have come to see — or to see more clearly — what I am documenting. And as the situations came into sharper focus, so I hope the language to describe them. On the other hand, in writing about how patient care should be, blame my choices on my optimistic belief, resilient despite repeated disappointment, that humanity inexorably improves.

I finished writing these essays in 2017 from inside the U.S. healthcare industry, drawing from observations during training in Perú and training and practice at Mayo Clinic in the United States. Yet, in my travels and my presentations, I have witnessed how the case they make resonates globally, regardless of how healthcare is organized, funded, or delivered. For these essays to remain valuable beyond the strictly contemporary, I have steered clear of the specifics of healthcare reform in the U.S. — the debates on whether everyone should have care disguised as debates on how to give everyone care — or I would have written only about them. The success of my work, however, must be judged on its ability to shape a revolution's language, thoughts, and actions, here and now, elsewhere and otherwise.

The privilege of the bedside has granted me access to stories, most of which I did not know I was carrying until I sat with a blank page. Anyone who knows me knows of my limited powers of recollection, so these stories, to surface, had to fight hard against the immediate, urgent, and noisy. I did not set out to write a book of stories, but I respect their power and put up little resistance when they insisted on being shared. Some of these stories came from conversations with family, peer clinicians, patients and their caregivers, and research colleagues. Unless I received their permission, I jumbled specifics where necessary to avoid recognition, to render the stories fictional but not false. I tried to protect their truth, their intimate genesis, and the privacy of their protagonists. I hope I have honored their beauty and served as a trustworthy conduit.

My goal is to persuade you that we must transform healthcare from an industrial activity into a deeply human one, capable of providing careful and kind care for all. To move toward careful and kind care, my strategy is to convey what makes industrial healthcare a profoundly undesirable development in society and how it contrasts with scientific, unhurried, and person-centered care. The difference between *what is* and *what should be* provides voltage to a revolution. This is why we revolt.

I don't expect the first spark of change to come from within, so I am banking on the public, on patients, to lead it. I have no doubt that students of the helping professions and health professionals of every sort, clinicians, will follow. I leave it to smarter people to invent and realize the specific actions that can bring about and sustain this patient revolution. My goal is that these pages will find a useful place on the table or the bookshelves of teams of revolutionaries, its language permeating through their own writing, speaking, thinking and, ultimately, action.

At the end, I hope you will join a patient revolution. Your actions may change the care you and your family receive, or the patient care for your entire community, or transform healthcare from an industrial activity to a human one. I hope to see you closing this book, rising, mobilizing, and persuading, with this book as the catalyst for your new role. I dream that its words, insufficient but necessary, arm you with the analyses, arguments, and actions you will need to revolt.

Part One

Cruelty

It was late at the premier teaching hospital in the country, and we were overworked and overwhelmed. Those patients in most trouble had made it in, but many waited outside, a domino line from the threshold of the emergency room to the edge of the hospital. Those inside were on gurneys in the treatment areas. They were in the hallway, on chairs, or on the floor. It was the era of hyperinflation and terror in Lima, Perú. I was one year away from graduating from medical school.

A corpulent and inebriated man came in with a large scalp laceration. One of my colleagues began to clean the wound. She misjudged that he would not need local anesthesia. He responded abruptly and violently, taking a bottle with some colored antiseptic solution and hurling it at her head, missing narrowly. Her scream and the red vitreous splash everywhere acted as the Bat-signal. Other doctors in training came rushing to her treatment bay. They first tried to restrain him. Soon, the gang in white coats was holding him down and beating him up. When it was over, the man had the original laceration and the swollen, bruised, and cut face the class of 1995 gave him.

What that patient received in punches, we delivered verbally to anyone who complained and whom we chose not to ignore. This was our emergency room, and these people, the patients, were here to bother us, to interrupt us, to make our day more difficult. We dehumanized the "laceration," the "foreign body," or the "appendix" without seeing the destitute and illiterate patients behind those labels. These subhumans were not only unfortunate and fortuneless but, in our eyes, were also careless, irresponsible, and stupid. Like a potent drug, equal parts efficacy and bitter pill, our emergency room could save a life while demeaning it.

Decades of psychological and sociological research explain the behavior of this white-coated mob. But what about the hospital rounds led by senior clinicians? A student six years my senior wrote a graduation thesis in which he noted that these rounds, when at the patient's bedside, almost never acknowledged the patient's existence: no greeting, small talk, explanations, nor elicitation of worries. Perhaps a question, but its purpose was to solve the diagnostic puzzle. Perhaps an exam, but it was to detect a sign. The patient as object, the subject barely noticed.

Yet, no one told us we, the trainees, were lacking in care. We ran a complex system of redistribution by which we asked more affluent patients to bring extra supplies that we would store and use to help poorer ones. We would use one patient's social assistance card to get free supplies for another who narrowly failed to meet the program's requirements. Thanks to this work, patients received tests, treatments, and operations; they got better and went home; and we received recognition. Perhaps we cared, but frankly, most of our work was completed to impress our senior residents and attending physicians with our resourcefulness and efficiency.

Occasionally, this churning would be interrupted. Mostly at night, when the hospital was quiet and slow. A sudden frameshift. An abrupt double take. The clinician suddenly noticing the person in the patient. A chair pulled. A chat.

Lines thrown from one boat to another. Permission to board.

"Who came to visit you today? Who is in that picture at your bedside?"

For an instant, the boats approached, abutted, and their wakes kissed.

Soon, they must diverge, drift, and sail away.

The clinician stands up as a new admission, a "pneumonia," rolls in.

Elsewhere in the Peruvian hospital, the lab receptionist was sipping his coffee, mixed with the exact amount of milk. Earlier he had filled a bucket with the tubes he discarded because they did not contain the exact amount of a patient's blood required for a test.

"No, no! The patient was a tough stick!" a trainee cried.

The lab receptionist remained unperturbed. The sample was lost, the test not run, and the intern looked bad on rounds. Sometimes the samples of several patients were lost or discarded because they came in seconds after the deadline. The man sipped his coffee, satisfied that his exacting work elevated the quality of the laboratory. The intern back at the bedside explained, "I am sorry. I have to draw your blood again." The cruelty of the protocol, rigidly applied.

On the other side of the world, 18 years later, I met the foremost American diabetes expert. He prescribes the latest medicines. He must do so, he says, because when he goes to meetings or colleagues consult him, he is expected to have experience with the latest advances and technologies. Thus, his patients are among the first to receive just-approved drugs. Pharmaceutical representatives know this, so they hand him glossy brochures about new medications. He is also often invited to speak at conferences about the experience he has accrued with these drugs.

Once, he and I coincided at a diabetes conference in India. One could easily see the addictive allure of his position. He was treated to luxurious events with guests from the Bollywood scene. At the end of his competent presentation, the host asked the audience to "stand up for a standing ovation." He left in a black stretch limo. In his talk, he had recommended that local clinicians use treatments with a cost and burden difficult to justify based on existing research. These clinicians, believing his pitch or, perhaps, hoping for his status, will switch their patients, like those of the American guru but much poorer, to the latest drugs. The cruelty of fame.

Back at home, it was time for my patient to refill a prescription. For the pharmacy to refill that prescription, however, the request must be made within 10 days of the previous fill running out. But the patient remembered to call too early, 11 days before the refill was needed. The system fails the stress test of kindness. "I cannot save your request and process it tomorrow ... you need to call again tomorrow." She forgot. A few weeks later, the patient explained to me why she did not take all the medicines. "My condition seems out of control now," she said. Everyone was just doing their job. The cruelty of our routines. The cruelty of petty rules.

In the news, I learn of a hospital's accounting department that has partnered with an agency to collect outstanding bills in full. The agency prioritizes the accounts by amount and likelihood of a successful collection. Agents knock door after door, threatening and harassing destitute families, some still mourning the permanent disability or death of their loved one. Some of these families had already worked with hospital representatives on a formula to pay their outstanding bills. "Our records do not reflect that," the collectors say, "and we will go to the end to get our money back." The cruelty of cold cash.

In other news, a CEO announced to his board that the generic drug they just acquired will have a price adjustment of several thousand percent. Their monopoly on this "market" firmly in hand, he is moving to cash in on behalf of the stockholders. In 2016, this scene replayed in the stories of daraprim, epinephrine auto-applicators, digoxin, naloxone, and other generics. Blame was allocated to the Food and Drug Administration, or FDA, (for enforcing regulation that slows the approval of generics), to lawmakers (for not regulating pharma's profits), to company boards (for placing beneficence far behind profits), to payers (for not negotiating drug prices, including Medicare, the U.S. public payer forbidden by law to negotiate them), and to CEOs (for doing anything for their performance bonuses). The consequences were allocated to patients, pricing people out of the treatments they needed and increasing the cost of healthcare for everyone else through hikes in insurance premiums. The cruelty of greed.

Cruelty seems to require that we, as clinicians, dehumanize patients, consider them not like us, not our kin. That we treat their suffering and dependent selves as a subspecies, as an extreme form of "them" with nothing in common with our humanity. Nothing in their name, their appearance, or their circumstance is able to bridge their distance from us. They are beds, diagnoses, samples, case numbers, or statistics. The expression in their eyes, the warmth of their heart despite their impossible circumstances, and the picture she keeps by her bedside of her granddaughter in a faraway city are all desperate gestures reaching for the reset button to make one human notice another.

Cruelty requires policies and procedures that discourage people, even the kindest, from noticing. One set of such policies defines jobs very narrowly. I get paid to do this, not to worry about the design limitations of a system in which I am no more than a replaceable part, a part that will be replaced if I don't do what I am expected to do. I am just following orders. Policies that retain professionals who become uninterested in the concrete downstream consequences of their actions on individual people, and thus behave unprofessionally.

Cruel policies affect how the work is done. Impossibly busy appointment schedules and heavy patient loads force clinicians, even the kindest, to see patients as a blur, noticing nothing particular about any of them. Policies that place vast distance between the administration and the hospital ward, between the receptionist and the bedside, between the decision-maker and the petitioner. This is a distance from which Ana, Jose, and Susan cannot be distinguished from each other or from other patients, all of them solidly "them."

These policies, motivated by the same industrial justifications, often dehumanize not only the patients but also those who are supposed to serve them and help them heal, even the kindest. The dehumanization of clinicians makes them expendable and interchangeable, like lightbulbs. Lightbulbs that, as the cruel system is finding out, can also burn out. And burned out clinicians and staff manifest a key deficit: the inability to respond to the suffering of a fellow human with empathy. Cruelty incites cruelty.

And yet, amidst incidents of cruelty, we find accidents of care. A nurse stayed after her shift to help her elderly hospital patient use his laptop to witness via live video his granddaughter's graduation. On her way home, a pharmacist took the box of medicines for a sick child traveling in Germany to the main office of the courier company after the prescription missed the last courier pickup truck. Five days after operating on his hip, the surgeon brought a chair he had at home to the patient's hotel room to make it easier for him to take a shower. Humans recognizing each other as fellow humans, disappointing what others expect of them, overcoming fear and violating the care protocols to make room for care, eschewing reputation in favor of a moment of intimacy that no one had to notice.

The antidote to cruelty is in the humanity of clinicians who, in a moment, remember why they went into health care. It is in rejecting the tendency of industrial healthcare to cause cruelty and to make each one of us capable of realizing our infinite potential to be cruel to others. It is in policies that make noticing each other the easiest thing to do. It is in creating space and opportunity for us to realize our equally infinite human potential to care for and about each other.

The "pneumonia" that rolled in? That is Ms. Seminario. The picture used as wallpaper on her smartphone? That is of her oldest daughter, Carmen. Ms. Seminario is afraid, short of breath, alone. She dreams of getting better so she can resume her life and embark on an often-postponed new quest. She is getting better for her children.

The clinician leans forward, unhurried.

Lines thrown, closer.

His eyes instantaneously sign a one-clause contract: "We are here now, for you and your care only."

He questions and gets answers. They make answers.

Boats moored together. Permission to board.

Unhurried touch. Examined. Reassured.

With cruelty always a possibility, for a moment, care happens.

Blur

I waited at the gate until all the passengers had deplaned. Amidst the crew came the captain of the commercial flight who had taken me and 128 other passengers on an A319 Delta flight from Minneapolis to Boston.

The idea of asking the pilot one question arose from a conversation I had with a leader in quality improvement. As is often the case, he used the analogy of healthcare as commercial air travel. This analogy compares the safety record of airlines and the methods by which they achieve it with healthcare's alleged ability to kill one jumbo jet worth of people every day. People like to point out that the analogy breaks down when one considers that, in contrast to doctors and their patients, the pilot shares outcomes with the passengers, particularly when the plane crashes. But my colleague brought up the pilot with an unexpected twist, "Victor, what we need is the experience that reliable airlines offer their passengers. Do you care who the pilot is when you board a plane?"

This was an interesting question. My mother grew up around planes. My maternal grandmother was among the first women to fly a plane in South America. My maternal grandfather was a hydroplane pilot with the Peruvian Air Force and served as a military attaché in Washington, D.C., during World War II. My mother was able, from an early age, to join the jet set and fly, years before quality and reliability were all but guaranteed to the level expected and achieved today. These early experiences have stayed with her. Today, when she flies, she is not comfortable until she verifies lots of grey hair on the captain. While flying, she listens to the engine and keeps her window shade up, interrogating the skies to predict and prepare for turbulence. It is difficult to be relaxed when traveling with her. She had learned that the pilot (and the co-pilot, the technicians that last checked the plane, and others) mattered.

That is a very different experience from mine. I travel more than I would like and as a result find myself flying in planes piloted by men and women who are barely more than voices on the PA. They report on the plane's altitude, the flight path, the expected arrival time, and the weather at our destination. They invite us to sit back, relax, and enjoy the flight. As I stood on the jet bridge, the anonymous professional behind this voice was about to be revealed; I was going to meet the pilot of my Minneapolis-Boston flight.

He (yes, Mom, tall and gray-haired), looked tired as he walked out of the tunnel. He had stood outside his cockpit as people were deplaning, thanking every one of the 128 passengers for flying Delta and wishing them a great day. He had shared some polite laughs with a few who cracked a joke or made a casual remark. After some pleasantries, I asked him, "Did any of the passengers catch your attention?" He slowed his pace and looked at me briefly, "No, not really. At the end of the day they are all a blur."

A blur.

I had a perfectly reliable flight, arrived safely and on time, piloted by systems, procedures, and a gray-haired pilot for whom the passengers had become a blur. Passengers, other than my mother, did not need to care about who the pilot was anymore. And the pilot did not need to care who the passengers were either. And this, air travel, was the analogy my quality improvement expert colleague was using to advance a new vision for healthcare!

A colleague of mine works as a physician in the Peruvian social insurance system, in which, impossibly, he is expected to see more than 30 patients in a morning. "What hurts? Let me see. Could be your liver. Take this treatment for now, go get this test, and make another appointment when you get the results. Next!"

Another colleague works at a cardiovascular clinic in Dalian, China. Snaking from the hallway, her patient queue comes into her office and right up to her desk. The next patients stand single file behind the one who sits across from her at the desk. All listen attentively to the exchange and, occasionally, ask questions and participate in the consultation of their otherwise unrelated comrade.

Patient care looks like this when a healthcare system, desperate to meet huge needs with scarce resources, underinvests in the supply of care, fails to educate the demand for care, and is marred by corruption and disregard for patients and frontline professionals. When I asked the Chinese cardiologist about her patients, she made a movement with her hand, the one you would make to describe fast cars on a highway. Yes, her patients were a blur.

A blur.

There are obvious circumstances in which caring for blurry patients is practically the only possibility, as it is for my colleagues from the understaffed systems in Perú or China and for those who heroically serve people crowded in refugee camps and mass casualty accidents.

Indeed, in these settings, focusing on a patient too long may rob care from others. When conditions are constrained not by necessity but by incompetence, greed, and corruption, caring for blurry patients can erode the moral and professional fabric of the system and of its professionals. Under these conditions, in which some profit at the expense of the despair of many, clinicians can become callous, angry, cynical, and incapable of empathy. This feeling is contagious, spreading upwards and across the administrative hierarchy. Without respite, everyone stops caring.

But patient blur is the mutable result of human choices, not the inevitable consequence of natural laws. To see the patient in his or her individuality, the clinician must appreciate the content and context of the patient's situation and how they relate to each other. Things said, implied, and gestured must be acknowledged, half-blurted lines and depressed murmurs pursued. This patient, here and now, is the one the clinician must notice clearly. To treat people with respect, clinicians must see patients not as blurs, but as sharply focused individuals in high definition.

Seeing each person in high definition does not mean having full knowledge about a person. This, I believe, is unattainable. It does not require the elimination of otherwise unavoidable ambiguity and uncertainty but rather their integration into care. Seeing patients in high definition requires more information about the patient, but it is not yet clear that this information must come from obsessive self-measurement of bodily functions or from the assessments of genes, proteins, or gut bacteria. Rather, I think sufficient details can be gleaned from simply noticing what is humanly and practically available.

The patient as the problem

Noticing prevents the avoidable ignorance that plagues decisions in fast medicine. By failing to address the patient situation, these hasty decisions fuel the need for additional tests and visits. Thus, one way to reduce the queue — at least the contribution of unwarranted return visits — and to support focused visits, that is, to avoid blur, is to treat people carefully the first time, every time. Reducing demand for patient care in this manner may powerfully stand against the tendency of industrial healthcare to degrade patients into what Isaiah Berlin called a "featureless amalgam."

Other ways to reduce demand for care make access to care tortuous (through insufferable and impersonal phone triage lines) or unaffordable (through high-deductible insurance schemes). Consider primary care phone lines designed to triage patients to the correct response: a clinic appointment, a call back from a nurse, a visit to the emergency department, or some other approach. The patient needs to get through the hold music to a nurse, who is often unfamiliar with the patient despite an ongoing relationship with the practice. Patients must answer an exhausting array of questions. Frustratingly, the patient's own primary care team would know the answer to many of these. Some patients delay proper care because they learn to avoid calling the line, give up partway through the lengthy call, or find the triaging result unsuitable. For them, the clinic's efficiency tool sets up a substantial barrier to care.

Payers can also reduce demand. High-deductible insurance schemes aim to further the distance between people and low-value care (which is a problem when care is of low value to payers and other parties, but necessary and desirable for patients). In this way, barriers to care represent inelegant solutions in the service of industrial goals based on the unkind and disrespectful notion of the patient as the problem.

The doctor will notice you now

Another way of reducing demand for patient care is to "make" fewer patients. Poverty, injustice, income inequality, violence (including adverse childhood events such as physical and psychological abuse), and alienation contribute to chronic stress, limited ability to enact healthy lifestyles, and poor access to preventive care. Together, these conditions increase the number of people, particularly among the disadvantaged, who go on to live with chronic ailments, such as obesity, diabetes, high blood pressure, chronic pain, and depression. Changing the unfavorable ecology of disadvantage through the political process is a major challenge for humanity, and also a just way to reduce the number of patients and their demand for health care.

Also, training people, as they become chronic patients, to self-care effectively may reduce their need for doctor visits. Self-care may promote health, whenever health is understood as the ability to adapt, self-manage, and thrive. Developing dependencies on clinicians is not consistent with this view of health, and thus fostering some distance between clinicians and patients may be both necessary and desirable. But that distance should result not from administrative decisions or policies but from understanding the patient situation, deciding together what distance is pertinent, and supporting patients in their self-care.

Alternative models of care can also reduce demand for individual patient appointments. Clinicians could use telemedicine to help homebound patients and those living in remote locations. Clinicians could also care for patients in small group visits, unhurried consultations in which patients also benefit from peer patient experience and support.

When patients need individual appointments, health care must respond kindly. Patients who take part in in-person office visits must capture the clinician's attention. To see the patient in high definition, multitasking clinicians must turn their attention away from the computer and ignore its demands for more data. Service technologies and other innovations, e.g., scribes or data collection using sensors without human input, could be designed to place industrial processes, such as documentation and billing, in the background. In turn, they can shift human processes to the foreground, helping clinicians develop a productive appreciation of and interaction with each patient. These efficiencies are not self-serving; they serve the work of care. There is so much more to learn about how to make patient encounters meaningfully helpful, within a sensible duration, and in the context of ongoing therapeutic relationships.

Before care for people and their lives becomes possible, we must rebel against the industrial healthcare's sickening trick, the illusion that the "who" is irrelevant, interchangeable. Each careful visit, a rejection of this trick; each high-definition encounter, an act of defiance.

Greed

To understand the mission of healthcare, we must infer it from its actions. What is healthcare trying to do? To what purpose does it invest its resources? What does it call success? Hospitals and clinics announce their quarterly financial performance and celebrate the expansion of their market share. These healthcare companies carefully manage their placement in the rankings published by trade magazines, engineer their patient online ratings, and optimize payers' "value" ratings. Short-term achievements of their industrial and financial activities produce bonuses for healthcare executives. Improving patient care outcomes, an assessment that would require lifting their gaze to the long-term horizon, does not. When they do lift their gaze, however, it is to assess market opportunities and where competitors are going. Healthcare has shifted its focus from patient care and instead has honed in on achieving goals that are industrial and financial.

Healthcare is focused on money. Managers often use this phrase to justify this priority: *No money, no mission*. While one could understand this in for-profit healthcare companies, it's also standard behavior

in many not-for-profit healthcare corporations. A focus on money
— greed — drives industrial healthcare away from patient care. To
deal with greed and to advance patient care, we must discover and
advocate for the antithesis of greed.

A devastating tornado in 1883 revealed the limited resources available in Rochester, Minnesota, to deal with the infirm. The Sisters
of St. Francis responded by deciding to build a hospital. When they
tried to recruit Dr. William W. Mayo to their efforts, he demanded
first that money be raised to build the facility. *No money, no mission.*
Making patient care their priority, the nuns raised the money and
opened Saint Marys Hospital. Over the next few decades, Dr. Mayo
and his two sons revolutionized the practice of medicine and surgery. Mayo Clinic was born — money just a means to achieve their
noble end.

Patient care organizations must exhibit business discipline to ensure
they have enough resources to be both sustainable and innovative.
In this way, these organizations can continue to pursue their mission and respond to the evolving needs of those for whom they care.
Business discipline is essential: no money, no mission. This phrase,
however, has a different and corrupting meaning for the healthcare
industry: money has taken over as the industry's *raison d'être* such
that patient care should happen only where it makes business sense.
Money has shifted from a resource for patient care to the product
of healthcare.

The language of healthcare, beyond "no money, no mission,"
uncovers this corruption of purpose. "Medical loss ratio" is how
payers describe the proportion of their income "lost" in paying for
patient care. "Risk" is how much of their reimbursement healthcare companies spend on caring for people. Healthcare executives,
like most humans, are wired to avoid loss and reduce risk; this
language signals the need to avoid and reduce patient care to make

money: less mission, more money.

There are innovations that avoid care or facilitate access to the supposedly appropriate level of care, drive efficiency, and lower costs to payers. Examples include "nonvisit" care provided through phone calls from nurses one has never met, "self-care" including self-testing and self-management, and "care delivery" by under-paid community health workers often lacking adequate training and support. These approaches advance mission while saving or making money. The money saved pays for robotic surgeries and proton beam radiation facilities. Such technologies contribute to the recruitment, retention, and ego of medical entrepreneurs, often photographed next to their latest acquisition. These, in turn, con-tribute to marketing efforts that expand market share and crush the competition and, for now, are better reimbursed by payers than primary care visits. Where there is more money, healthcare com-panies find more missions.

Most people with unglamorous chronic conditions, conditions that cause pain or insomnia or that cause dysfunction that cannot be medically explained or surgically fixed, will find themselves in the discarded bin of "no money, no mission." Caring for these patients clogs the pipelines and distracts healthcare companies from their more profitable missions. In this healthcare industry, some patients — the ones who bring in the dollars — are more worthy of care than others.

In pursuing short-term financial gains, the healthcare industry has corrupted its mission. It has stopped caring. Experts can debate myriad explanations for this situation. And yet, to fix it, we must understand what fuels it. And it is this: greed.

Trapped between seduction and frustration

At the end of my medical internship, I was assigned to a three-month rotation in the hospital of a mining camp nested in the Peruvian Andes. The camp's hospital was well-resourced and well-run. Its patients were miners, administrative staff, and their families. Healthcare was part of the compensation plan of the miners, and some used it excessively.

The demand for services caught my fellow interns and me — youngsters with minimal prior experience — unprepared. We reacted in a rigorously academic way. We decided to stop the practice of prescribing steroid injections to help patients overcome common colds. This practice had started a few years back. Whoever came up with it had shown a wild disregard for the side effects of this remedy — suppression of the immune system and worsening of diabetes, to name two — while exploiting the common belief that injectable medicines were more potent.

These injections were remarkable: With one stab people could leave the emergency department feeling treated, a dream for a tired intern. But not for the Universidad Peruana Cayetano Heredia interns, the wise saviors from Lima! Patients, trained by their prior visits to the emergency room to want more than what they need, complained that we had taken away the shots. Labor representatives interpreted our righteous therapeutic restraint — acetaminophen and plenty of water — as the manifestation of a new company policy. They threatened one of the largest copper mines in the world with a strike if healthcare benefits were cut. After the dust settled, we, the interns, had been responsible for a temporary increase in the world price of copper.

As in the Andes, patients can respond to healthcare messages by driving up the consumption of healthcare while some parts of the system expect them to behave thriftily. For example, healthcare often markets lucrative and imprecise screening tests of no value to people. Findings from these tests require additional, often lifelong, healthcare. For instance, the anxious young person who sought care for chest pain and received a coronary stent inserted "to be safe" on a "borderline" obstruction seen on a "definitive" coronary angiogram obtained "just in case" after an otherwise normal stress test. This unsuspecting victim — coronary stents don't help people without chest pains and don't prevent people from having or dying from heart attacks — would go on to gratefully receive care from a cardiologist and take anti-clotting and cholesterol-lowering medicines for years. A healthy person turned into a lifelong patient and a paying customer. "They saved my life," he would say, strengthening the word-of-mouth campaign.

Marketing advertises to patients the latest irresistible innovations. The ads do not present arguments based on research evidence — few if any drug or device ads directed at consumers present the impact of these innovations in terms that people can consider and compare with alternatives. The impact of these innovations on outcomes that matter to patients is not discussed. Will this help me avoid premature death, mitigate my suffering, or preserve or recover my function? Instead, the ad shows people miraculously running through green fields, celebrating their unrealistically healthy happiness, the voice actor inviting you to "ask your doctor about ..." This "experience" is the selling argument for the test or treatment, as if it was deodorant or a vacuum cleaner. The healthcare industry has argued that direct-to-consumer advertising is education for the public while offering a hyped sales pitch that plays unashamedly to the gullibility of uninformed users, and plays both with their fears and their hopes.

In these and other ways, the healthcare industry fabricates patient wants, and then uses these patients' search for what they believe will be best for them to satisfy its own needs. These industrial actors satisfy their greed by promoting maximal healthcare spending. Yet, there are other actors, such as insurers and other payers, who satisfy their greed by promoting minimal healthcare spending. The patient is caught between these two: seduced by the former, frustrated by the latter.

Payers demand restraint from consumers. They ask patients to compare prices, to shop around, and to find the best value. Rather than recognize the difficulty of behaving like a savvy consumer in the healthcare bazaar, payers assume patients to be irresponsible and demand upfront payments to make sure they have "skin in the game." High deductibles, high premiums, and high co-pays act as walls that keep patients — the enemy, the risk, the loss — away. This is particularly the case when out-of-pocket expenses compete, and often lose, against rent, food, security, education, or recreation. These walls act as indiscriminating barriers that patients must overcome to reach the care they need. Efforts patients must make to jump over or break through these barriers compete with the work necessary to enact the routines of much-needed self-care. Those who have no choice but to postpone or stop accessing care, or cease taking prescribed medicines, don't get help to minimize the burden of treatment. They are labeled instead as noncompliant.

Payers may justify these practices in their roles as stewards of limited resources seeking to reduce their use on interventions of low value to patients. Yet, clinicians will prescribe and affluent patients will access these services, suggesting to those left out that this care is indeed valuable and desirable — like fashionable shoes and fast cars. Suffering then results from not being able to afford the care you think you need or from receiving it until you can no longer afford it. Suffering also stems from the sacrifices made to receive unnecessary care you were told you needed, and from having care, necessary or not, denied to you even as you saw others get it. In contradiction with its ideal intent, industrial healthcare alleviates *and* causes suffering. In these streets of confusion, contradiction, and aggression, in the shadows of life, the sick wander. The only light intermittently breaking the shadow is coming from a flashing neon sign, sometimes on, sometimes off: "More healthcare is better."

Pay the doctor with a guinea pig

We should be able to trust clinicians to protect patients from being miscast and manipulated as mere consumers. This term, clinician, describes anyone who is privileged enough to stand at the bedside of those who suffer. From that privileged position, clinicians can offer competent and compassionate care, and communities have always rewarded them for it. The daughter of one of the managers was visiting the mining camp in which I worked as an intern when she went into labor. By noon the next day, her father, now the grateful grandfather of a healthy boy, had assembled a long table featuring the delicacy of the area, roasted guinea pig. Oh, and plenty of beer. He successfully insisted that the doctor (in training) should enjoy the fruits of his labor, while the first-time grandfather enjoyed the fruits of his daughter's. Beer and gratitude flowed.

Over the last 60 years in the United States, there has been an evolution in the way clinicians are paid, with some specialists earning exorbitant incomes. The recipients of this windfall offer a list of justifications for their wealth: long years of income-forgoing training, large debt at graduation, risk of litigation, cost of malpractice insurance, and ability to bring big money to the coffers of clinics and hospitals by conducting complex procedures. Indeed, many of these clinicians found fame in outperforming their peers and, in the process, becoming exorbitantly rich.

Not all clinicians, however, pursue the path of individual entrepreneurship and wealth. Over 150 years ago, clinicians got together to form multispecialty clinics. These clinics compensated clinicians via salaries; salaried clinicians made the same money regardless of the number of procedures they practiced or referrals they made to colleagues or tests — no kickbacks, no bonuses. Isolated from profit motives, patients may find the recommendations of salaried clinicians to undergo or forgo tests and treatments more trustworthy.

Linking a proportion of a clinician's compensation to the number of patients or procedures (also called volume), to the documented "quality of care" given, or to the money spent in patient care introduces biases against careful and kind care. While the intention may be to ensure sufficient productivity from clinicians, income that depends on volume of work can turn each patient into an economic opportunity, an anonymous money-making blur. In part, this explains why there are more surgeries where there are more surgeons compared to adjacent areas with similar needs but fewer surgeons. This is why when a new gynecologic surgeon moves into town, we can expect more hysterectomies, beyond patient need or want. In a pay-for-volume system, this may very well be why the hospital hired the gynecologic surgeon! Researchers have described this situation as one in which supply of a service induces demand for that service.

Linking income to the complexity or completeness of the documentation of care focuses the clinician's attention on documenting. Facilitated by electronic health records optimized to improve financial compensation, clinicians produce heaps of notes. More notes, more money. These records poorly communicate what is going on to other clinicians, to the same clinician, and to the patient, despite being voluminous. Like a mistuned radio station, the documents are noise rich, but signal poor. These records are filled with default auto-populated notes about organs that felt normal although they were never examined. Cutting and pasting efficiently adds detail to notes, introducing errors that give smooth prostates to women and declined vaginal exams to men. In these records, the fully described patient remains a ghost, a blurry outline covered in confused and unimportant detail. When they have been harnessed, these imperfect records have, however, made important contributions to the statistical functions of healthcare, including research and quality improvement. And, amidst the noise, one can often find notes that say something meaningful, messages in the bottle floating in a sea of information.

Some old notes — scribbled before the electronic era — are unhelpful. Many cannot be read, but one does not need an hour to determine their low value. Others were artful works of synthesis in which clinicians reported insights they judged relevant for either their next visit with this patient or for the patient's next visit with another colleague. "The patient is improving. Worried about getting back to work. The incision is healing without evidence of infection. Will discharge in about 1 week if no complications." The modern note, more complete so that it can "support" better reimbursement, would need two pages to say more, and it may still not say as much. Documentation takes so much attention away from patients and so much time from the clinical encounters, half of it by some estimates, that it contributes to patient and clinician dissatisfaction. Why then would healthcare companies pay exorbitant figures for electronic medical records and hire scribes to attend to these records that support care so poorly? According to their sales brochures, healthcare companies that invest billions in the top record systems can demonstrate better financial performance. The answer is money.

Other policies have clinicians "sharing risk." In these schemes, clinicians make more money when they order fewer tests or referrals. This puts them on a collision course with consumers who come with their "Ask Your Doctor" ad in hand or demand a referral to a specialized service.

The robot will see you now

Some healthcare organizations, many of which are nominally not-for-profit, are involved in an arms race with a neighboring health-care company competing for more market share. They are willing to invest in and encourage patients to demand highly profitable care as they limit the offer and constrain the demand for less profitable tests and treatments. In this race, competitors place billboards and ads on TV driving people to demand their latest technological acquisitions or encouraging people onto the operating table of their just-arrived star surgeon or surgical robot. This feeds into the widely held belief that more healthcare, more sophisticated, more technologically advanced is better. However, many of these advances are placed in front of patients before there is research evidence of their usefulness.

Take robotic surgery. It is now the dominant way in which hyster-ectomies are performed in the United States. Surgeons who take the uterus out, usually because of benign masses or bleeding, were trained traditionally to do this through the vagina. This opera-tion does not leave a visible scar, has fewer complications, and the recovery is quicker than robotic surgery. This inexpensive opera-tion would seem better than the one conducted using a robot, a pro-cedure that leaves five visible scars, is more complicated, and costs more. Yet, in the U.S., robot-assisted surgery has quickly become the most common form of hysterectomy. Surgical programs now teach young surgeons to operate using the robot. Seeking the comfort of using the same state-of-the-art equipment in which they began to learn their art, freshly minted surgeons demand that a robot be pur-chased as a condition for employment. Patients in the community celebrate the acquisition of the new equipment and the hiring of the new surgeon. They will not know, however, how many of the 80 operations required to achieve proficiency the surgeon has completed. Patients in the community will experience avoidable complications as the surgeon operates his way up that learning curve. They will also be unaware of the need to cover the cost of buying and maintaining the robot with more operations. These factors act as a powerful incentive to find reasons to operate, where a medical treatment or watchful waiting could have done. The robot takes money; the robot makes money. The patient leaves money, time, and health ... and her uterus behind.

And the money flows upstream, to investors and executives. Many hospitals and clinics started as charities (some still bill themselves as nonprofits), but today most are healthcare companies. Some are large investor-owned corporations, with executive staff focused on distributing dividends from their profitable activities to their investors. Some are nonprofits dedicating an increasing proportion of their revenue to cover the cost of managing the organization rather than to advancing and sustaining its mission. Their chief executives must produce returns not just to sustain the organization and to pay for innovations but also to cover increasingly extravagant executive compensation.

The usual reason given to justify astronomical executive compensation is that these nonprofits must compete in the marketplace of executives. To get the best, they must be willing to pay for the best. This argument is used even when organizations have a long tradition of selecting its leaders from within. That these executives get performance bonuses for meeting short-term financial targets instead of improving patient care and outcomes undermines the appropriate mission and disconnects decisions from the care of patients. More money, more money; no money, no money. That they get bonuses even when patients have suffered from incompetent administration of their facilities is scandalous. More money, less mission.

Magical powers are attributed to competition, including improvements in service experience and lower prices. For many reasons, this is not often the case in healthcare. Rather, competitors will attract and find reasons to push patients through their services to achieve financial targets. When organizations in a community compete to serve patients, they may offer frivolous services, unlikely to help yet profitable. It is hard to be the best at "just right" when your competitor offers "more" and your investors demand better returns. And this applies to healthcare companies and payers. Fueled by greed, healthcare accounts for an increasingly large fraction of our economies, growing at a quicker pace than in countries in which tax-funded non-profit care is the norm. That the former also excludes millions from care, consumes more resources, and produces worse health outcomes than the latter compounds its limitations: your money *and* your life.

Dawkins' tree analogy is helpful here. In nature, competition has made trees grow taller as they reach for the sun. Getting more sun means more energy, which in turn is spent growing taller. At the base, some plants unable to grow are overshadowed and die. Other trees get in on the competition for sunlight. If these trees could agree to grow to a certain height, one in which they all could get enough sun, they could save enormous energy (and need less of it). But trees have not evolved language, civilization, communities, or a sense of justice. We need healthcare companies that behave better than trees.

What the market can bear

The money does not come directly from the pockets of the sufferer because, almost always, someone else pays. That "someone else" turns out to be all of us — either by paying increasingly higher insurance premiums or via the swallowing up of increasingly high proportions of public budgets. This renders the link between human suffering and exorbitant prices for drugs and devices indirect and invisible.

"Visionary" drug company leaders seek to meet stockholder expectations by setting very high prices for their drugs. They decide to charge these prices even for drugs long past their already very generous patent protection period, long after paying for the cost of development and producing copious profits. Their justification? The market — not the invisible hand, but the system built by prescription benefit managers, health insurers, lobbyist, and conflicted regulators — is willing or able to pay.

Medicines that arguably cure hepatitis C are sold at $1,000 per tablet. The argument for this? The market can pay this charge. This cost, they argue, matches the cost of care for end-stage liver disease and liver transplant, which are now avoided in the fraction of patients who would have progressed to that point. You must pay for value, they say. So, if the drug is useless, you should pay less; if the drug is effective, you should pay more. Why, this one cures! If a drug is lifesaving, we should be ready to pay the highest prices. Think of antibiotics, antivenom sera, rehydration solutions, or oxygen. These can be lifesaving when used in extreme situations. To charge exorbitant prices for them forces a decision: your money or your life. How much you and your family are willing to pay to access lifesaving treatments, the size of the ransom, should not determine their price. This is not healthcare, but extortion.

Pharmaceutical and medical device corporations also oversee the evaluation of their own innovative products and pay regulators fees to get them approved. When huge profits are at stake and the size of those profits depends on beating the competition, anything goes. That explains their willingness to settle and pay large penalties rather than avoid fraudulent activities in favor of their products. No wonder the research intended to guide clinicians and calibrate user expectations is corrupt, almost always finding in favor of the sponsor's product and leading the marketing effort to increase market share.

Pay for performance

Large employers contract with health plans, private health insurers, and all sorts of other business to buy healthcare for their employees and beneficiaries. They want to see their money go further and have pushed for a model of value in healthcare, one that reduces the use of resources needed to achieve the best possible quality, safety, outcomes, and experience of care. Measurement of the outcomes of care is in its infancy, and first-generation measures are easy to assess but are largely disconnected from the quality of care patients experience. Some measures, such as quality of life, are hard to improve; others, such as the proportion of patients with diabetes with optimal blood sugar control, are easy to improve by excluding, firing, or selecting patients.

Yet the easiest way to improve value to a payer — care "delivered" per dollar paid — is to offer the same service to that payer for a lower price. At the extreme, this requires the healthcare company to adjust its "payer mix" (to reduce access to patients whose care is reimbursed by a stingy payer) or to give different care depending on who pays. Some patients experience less "love" from their healthcare companies when they turn 65 and become covered by Medicare, a reimbursement scheme designed to be stingy. As we discussed, some innovations, for instance nonvisit care, seek to keep patients like these from care, particularly from expensive care.

The antithesis of greed

As healthcare constrains its mission to save money, it allows waste and profits to steal resources for care. Healthcare should not waste precious resources or scarce talent that patients urgently need. Smarter regulation, appropriate technology, and quality improvements can all reduce waste. The savings from waste reduction must be applied to care. Greed should not extract these savings from the system to reward a few actors when the system needs to provide effective, evidence-based, efficient, safe, timely, equitable, and patient-centered care. Instead of leaving the system as take-home profits, these resources are needed to make top-quality care sustainable and to pay for innovations that meet the ever-changing requirements of those in need of care. We must confront the injustice of having some people go without care because of greed. We must find the antithesis of greed.

Maybe the antithesis of greed is moderation. Patients and families must recognize that it is not true that more healthcare is better. Not enough care is dangerous, but so is too much. Goldilocks care is essential. This requires judgment, seeing the situation of each patient in high definition and selecting judiciously the care that is needed and wanted, neither more nor less. Healthcare companies and corporations must own up to the extent to which their practices seek to price people out or limit access to people because of their (or their payer's) ability to pay. Then they must change these practices. Healthcare companies should not exclude people too sick to jump their hurdles. They should not seek money at the expense of their mission.

Alternatively, healthcare agents could pursue profits up to a point. Mission first, for money, but not too much. Clinicians would seek satisfying salaries, enough to stop them from seeking supplements outside of medicine or bonuses linked to volume or value. This would require reducing the burden of malpractice insurance and eliminating usurious student loans. These salaries should differ little from specialty to specialty to make sure the right people are in the right positions for the right reasons.

Healthcare companies would focus their resources to caring. Marketing and the technological arms race with other hospitals would be replaced with coordination with the community to meet its real needs. In Hamilton, Ontario, hospitals don't compete with each other. Rather, they offer care in a manner that makes the overall offer comprehensive, with no money wasted on advertising competing services or on setting up and maintaining duplicate and redundant services. To keep all the value in healthcare, all healthcare organizations should reinvest earnings into patient care (for instance, to extend the time patients and clinicians can spend together), including the training of professionals and the funding of the scientific backbone of patient care. Administrators seeking a career in healthcare would know they will do well financially, but exorbitant salaries and bonuses would no longer be part of their compensation.

This should also affect the production and commercialization of drugs and devices by corporations designed to achieve moderate profits. If a drug or device is a lifesaver or can profoundly affect the quality of life of a person, the public has an interest to make it widely and affordably available. This should be reflected in regulation (patent protection) and contracting (warrantied pricing and purchasing). On the other hand, payers may need to pay more for a drug or device that offers only a minor improvement, such as more convenient dosing.

Cures, antibiotics, vaccines, rehydration solutions, antivenom sera, and other essential medicines would be available for free to the end user. Those in charge of production and distribution would be allowed to make, at most, a moderate profit, enough to ensure sufficient and sustainable production and distribution. Intermediaries, even if they were to make minimum profits, contribute only to the end user's cost. Thus, every effort should be made to eliminate profit makers sandwiched between producers and buyers.

Some people believe that the only reason medicine moves forward is money — that competition and profits drive innovation. They believe money motivates brilliant people to go into basic science to discover cures; it is what makes people study medicine, nursing, therapy, or pharmacy; it is what keeps clinicians up at night on call or compels them to jump onto a helicopter amid a storm to retrieve a donated organ for transplantation.

I don't think so. Even when corporation-partnering universities, healthcare companies, venture capitals, and other industrial actors work to communicate these beliefs, even when they succeed in attracting a cadre of greedy people to a career in care, I stand with young idealistic people who enter health care to make a difference in the lives of others, often because of their own experience with disease and treatment. Moved by empathy, their passion focused on solving a big problem, their immense talent achieves great good for many. It is their mission, as it was the mission of those who came before them, who worked harder for less, when the need was more desperate and the treatments were fewer. It is their destiny, and I refuse to believe that the moderation in expectations of income would make them set the alarm an hour later or suggest they should stop experimenting after their ninth cup of coffee.

There is no natural law that commands corporations of any kind to place the interests of their stockholders and administrators first. A more natural law would state that if you meet or exceed the needs of your customers, if you respect the people you serve, if you don't lie to them or shortchange them in the quality of your offering, and if you don't extort them, their loyal business will follow. That your company is the only one offering that service or drug cannot justify exorbitant prices or low quality but rather calls for more responsibility. Yes, you can get away with it and regulation does not limit you (thanks to your powerful lobby), but your values should stop you from abusing people rendered desperate by illness or the employees you deploy to care for them. This will require regulation banning excessive profit seeking and a new class of healthcare leaders that are effective managers of the precious resources placed in their hands — the creativity, compassion, time, and dollars of health professionals, scientists, payers, and generous citizens.

Cortisone, one of the world's most effective medicines, was placed by Mayo Clinic in the hands of Merck Sharpe and Dohme for one dollar. To this day, almost 75 years later, the drug remains inexpensive and widely available. Yet, today, aggressive executives are buying makers of generic drugs and selling them for 1,000 times their prior sale price. Why? Because they can. There is nothing stopping them. Well, not true. What stopped Mayo and Merck from excessively profiting from their miraculous Nobel Prize-winning drug was the values of their people. Those values should not only permeate patient care but also the societal contracts and regulations that protect the interests of those who greed makes most vulnerable.

Values of careful and kind care, like a spirit that blows everywhere possible, can turn industrial healthcare into patient care. The patient revolution's activism must help this spirit blow further and deeper. It must moderate financial expectations. It must put patients first. It must pay for existing cures and new advances from the money saved from forgoing exorbitant profits and preventing waste. It must celebrate that these innovations are available to everyone who needs them, regardless of ability to pay.

Perhaps moderation is not the ultimate antithesis of greed. Perhaps we can uncover it in the notion of all being on the same boat, a notion that will ultimately serve to moderate financial expectations in healthcare. This notion of a common fate is core to our humanity, its integrity offended when one of us falls ill and cannot recover because another one plans to profit from his misfortune. Rather than simply moderation, an attenuation of the same instincts, what stands opposite to greed is solidarity. Rather than a reform of healthcare financing and profits, we need a revolution of care. In caring for each member of our kin, we see ourselves wounded; in responding to the needs of every single one of us, we see the possibilities of our action: lives unhindered by disease and treatment.

Burden

They get together for an hour and a half the third Monday of every month. They come to help us because they care, they want to give back, and they want to help others. Since 2004, the Patient Advisory Group has helped us at the Mayo Clinic's Knowledge and Evaluation Research Unit, or KER Unit. They come to teach us what it feels like to be patients, to help us develop our ideas about research, to be partners in conducting projects and reporting results. They are dedicated: 13 years later, they are still at it.

Marge was the group's hero. She had lived with diabetes for longer than anyone else. She had "in-your-face" diabetes — type 1. She wore an insulin pump all the time. She pricked her fingertips, at the painful junction of blood vessels and nerve endings, between sitting down and taking her first bite. Before each meal, she counted carbohydrates in her diet and considered what amount of insulin to use. She was meticulous. She was proud. And she seemed healthy after five decades of living daily with this routine. She showed up to the monthly meetings on time and in one physical and emotional piece. She smiled.

At one of these meetings of the Patient Advisory Group, the group discussed the burden of their treatments. We wanted to understand what these patients endured in order to live productive lives unhindered by diabetic complications, to have a chance for a long and healthy life, like Marge. They told stories of uncoordinated appointments and miscommunication, of false hopes and fads. Faces cringed as they remembered the doctors and nurses who belittled their expertise, threatened them with bad outcomes, and fired them when "they failed." They spoke of negotiating barriers, approvals, and permissions to get clinicians to share records and talk to each other. Of how hard they had to work to find useful and trustworthy information, or to keep up with appointments, bills, and medication refills. Of how, like in the movie *I, Daniel Blake*, patients must work alone through the system's "digital by default" set of impenetrable apps and web interfaces with their own "pencil by default" skills. And, of course, they all had to make the treatment of diabetes work within the demands of their everyday life.

Marge smiled. She had a wonderful doctor. The doctor always knew what Marge needed to do. And Marge always did it, before and after retiring from her nursing job. "Burden of this treatment? Nah! This is what I have to do to stay alive and well."

I pushed back, "So treatment does not interrupt your life? Not even sometimes?"

"No", she said.

As Marge was telling us about the harmonious symbiosis between her life and her diabetes treatment, she reached down to her purse. She did not retrieve anything. The discussion moved on to the work of refilling medications and of adjusting diabetes treatments to account for weddings and infections. Then she did it again. She reached into her purse, but nothing came out. Julia, another participant who was sitting next to her, noticed. Sweetly, subtly, she nudged Marge into checking her sugar levels. Marge hesitated, fruitlessly reaching for her bag again. Julia joined the search and found the sugar meter. By this time, everyone had noticed and the session had stopped. Marge's diabetes treatment, causing the low blood sugar reaction, had interrupted Marge, Julia, and the whole group.

At first, the body reacts violently to plummeting sugar levels: shaking, sweating, and a feeling of impending doom. Because the brain only uses sugar for fuel, tunneling and graying of vision and a decline in mental capacity follow. When patients, like Marge, have had diabetes for many years and experience low blood sugars with some frequency, they tend to lose those first fierce yet lifesaving symptoms. This leaves them vulnerable and in need of others — family, coworkers, teammates, strangers — to notice odd behavior, slurred speech, and inability to coordinate, to think and to act quickly to restore sugar levels.

Julia gave Marge glucose tablets. As the sugar levels rose, Marge became herself again and smiled. "What burden? This is what I have to do to stay alive with diabetes." And she did, living with diabetes for most of her inspiring life.

Did Marge have to experience episodes like this? Are these interruptions the price she must pay for the benefits of treatments? I've learned that, for now, the answer is a clear, frightening, yes. But it does not have to be.

Why I was drawn to understand the burden of our treatments was precisely this sense: that the work of patients and the interruptions of life required for treatment are an unavoidable part of being sick. Diabetes causes high blood sugars. Marge's low blood sugar reaction was a result of too much treatment, too much insulin. The treatment directly caused the interruption, not the disease. In fact, treatment disrupted her life in other ways, before every meal, every day. Marge would acknowledge as much, but not label these tasks as burdensome. She had adapted to her routine. She had lived with her disease for decades, its treatment her lifesaving companion. And, when her treatment interrupted her? It was as if Marge did not want to upset her treatment by calling it names.

This experience was in no way unique, as my colleague Dr. Kasia Lipska found out. When she published a brilliant op-ed in *The New York Times* criticizing the rocketing cost of insulin, she received many angry letters. She expected as much from the parties she had clearly identified as contributing to the problem: the pharmaceutical companies, the pharmacy benefits managers, regulators, and payers. She wanted better for patients, to reduce the financial burden of their treatments, and this meant making insulin more affordable for patients like Marge, who need insulin to live. So, it was particularly painful for her to receive angry letters from patients and patient organizations. These letters stung and burned her heart, leaving Dr. Lipska with the hollow and sickening feeling that she had somehow failed the people for whom she was advocating. These patient letters were laden with fear. They started by noting how insulins and their delivery devices — hair-thin needles, nifty pens, and automated pumps — had gotten better, easier to use, more effective, and safer. They worried that all this innovation — inching closer to an artificial pancreas, the organ that produces insulin — could be put at risk if the profits of these companies were curtailed by insisting on the affordability of insulin. One can hear them say between the lines, "What burden? This is what I have to pay to get the treatment I need to live."

The CEO of Eli Lilly and Company, a major manufacturer of insulin, acknowledged that insulin was getting more expensive but remarked that care for the complications of untreated diabetes was still more expensive. Competition among manufacturers has not reduced the cost of insulin as people sometimes expect in other "markets." Here, competition with the other insulin manufacturers has led to a relentless increase in price of all brands. Insulin manufacturers profit greatly, greedily, but so do pharmacy benefit managers, meddlers who extract fortunes from insulin transactions, and thus increase its price, in exchange for unclear service to insurers. Insulin makers may say, "Burden? This is what *our companies* must do to stay alive."

Patients are cutting back on other basic needs to afford their insulin program: food, clothing, housing, education, and recreation all must wait in line for leftover money. Patients are meeting in parking lots. In these impromptu markets, patients with an insulin surplus sell to those with a need. "Burden? This is what we need to stay alive."

The work of being a patient

The anxiety caused by increasingly unaffordable treatments, the financial and practical burdens of obtaining those treatments, plus the daily challenges that Marge, Julia, and other patients like them face to take care of their diabetes and other chronic conditions, contribute to the burden of treatment. It is not simply the time patients spend (and how they wish they could have spent it elsewhere) but also the emotional work, the frustrating hurt involved in accomplishing each task, made often so maddeningly difficult for no apparent reason.

Living with disease, with many diseases, is becoming increasingly demanding as industrial healthcare delegates medical errands to patients, tasks they must complete to receive timely and coordinated care. To improve the efficiency of brief clinic appointments, patients are being asked to complete forms and come prepared with questions, or to record the visit so that they can review clinician's explanations and instructions at their own speed. Access to the medical record, chock-full of jargon that screams "not written for you," comes with the expectation that patients will proofread it. With 80 percent of its content copy-and-pasted from previous notes, Ms. Jones' record may confidently describe her as fully employed a decade after she broke the piñata at her retirement party.

I encountered the work of being a patient early in my training. Hospitalized patients, lying patiently in their beds, were clearly not doing much, all the medical work in the hands of clinicians. But some of the work was not medical. In the national hospitals of Perú in the early 1990s, care was nominally free. Yet, families were asked to pay some and to bring supplies necessary for the care of their loved ones. Medical students, turned into entrepreneurial Robin Hoods, ran errands for these patients to secure unaffordable supplies, got someone else to pay for tests and procedures, and kept a stockpile of supplies. We would partner with families to get what was necessary; some families organized *polladas*, chicken dinner parties, to raise funds. Two decades later, as I contemplate the work my patients must do to cope and thrive, to keep their lives unhindered by illness, almost all that work — treatment and errands — is in the patient's hands.

Despite its importance, I don't recall a single lecture in my 14 years of training or know of a single chapter in any medical textbook about the work of patients. Every six months, my patients spend two to four hours in the clinic. In the other 4,316 hours, patients must figure out how to make self-care coexist harmoniously with life. To the clinic, and to anyone unwilling to look or ask, this work is invisible and silent. Furthermore, no healthcare company assesses how much work they give patients to do. Unaware of how burdened patients and families are, healthcare managers have proclaimed the patient "the most underutilized resource in healthcare." Not only is this declaration unpleasant, uncaring, and profoundly industrial, but it is also tragically ignorant of how implementing treatments and navigating healthcare overwhelm patients and families.

For the healthcare industry, patient work is not only invisible but also free. As industrial healthcare delegates more work to patients, it removes these costs from its balance sheet, appearing more efficient. For organizations that seek to optimize healthcare value, i.e., quality achieved per unit of cost, shifting work to patients makes their services "high value." Managers may celebrate that the work was delegated to an "engaged" person while freeing up scarce healthcare resources. A win-win situation in their books.

All this work takes effort, attention, and time, but limited research exists that uncovers how much this takes; current estimates place that time at two hours per day, a part-time job. Some patients with one medical condition in a stable psychosocial situation may perhaps be able to accommodate all these delegated medical errands into whatever else is going on in their life. Its to-dos can be neatly listed between the urgent and the important, among the demands from family, work, and community. These can be crossed off during the time they might otherwise set aside for quiet rest, woodworking, dreaming, planning, adventure, naps, or conversation.

But it is not only the time spent on patient work but also the hardship involved in accommodating this work while life goes on. Patients must respond to the demands, often more meaningful and urgent, that their lives make, such as having a baby, taking a job promotion, learning a new skill, having fun with friends, enjoying a concert in the park, or taking a relaxing walk on the beach. When life makes more dramatic demands, the struggle is much harder, as patients must make treatment work while they take care of loved ones who have fallen ill, while they look for a new job, while they make ends meet, or while they avoid eviction.

For most mortals, this accumulated work ends up simply being too much. More than 40 percent of people over 65 report that health-care gives them too much work. Many delegate the work to family members, but others — those who live alone, are unwilling or unable to ask for help, or live in poverty — simply do what they can and the rest gets postponed. Clinicians brand patients who do not implement the care plan with a label that, in my experience, is extremely difficult to shake off, a scarlet letter that describes not their circumstance but their character. They are noncompliant.

Noncompliance is more than a nasty label. It describes people who appear to understand what is asked of them but don't do it. Unreliable, irresponsible folks. They are not going to do well, and their avoidable complications will cost the system. I know my colleagues and I have received no training to care productively for patients with this label. Our protocols say nothing about how to help with the care that takes place at the kitchen table, the bathroom, the nightstand, the workplace, the insurance help line, the clinic phone bank, the website, the pharmacy queue, the bus stop, or the clinic hallway. Thus, clinicians who choose to work under the influence of productivity incentives — pay for performance schemes promising dollars for outcomes — will see the care of noncompliant patients as a money-losing, risky, and unrewarding proposition. Noncompliance is one of the leading causes that clinicians and healthcare companies cite for firing patients.

In this sea of impotence and incompetence, we assume noncompliant patients need more education, that their inability to execute instructions is surely the result of ignorance. Education is helpful when lack of expertise in self-care means that regimens can only be implemented as prescribed, rather than shaped to fit within life's routines. This shaping requires expertise to know how and when to make exceptions and cut corners in ways that keep the value of the program and make it more feasible. This kind of practical wisdom is often found in other expert patients, not in the class or in the bulleted facts of the educational pamphlet.

Others may think "noncompliant" patients need motivation, to change their behavior, or to become "empowered" or "activated." Incentives and penalties will "ensure people take responsibility for their lives." These tactics of education and motivation are frustratingly unhelpful for most overwhelmed patients. It is as if we keep screaming directions to the lost tourist in a language they still cannot understand.

Healthcare companies and their employees may get a hint if they were to notice. Very often, "noncompliant" patients are otherwise diligent and caring parents, employees of the month at two jobs they must keep, and active citizens and advocates for their neighborhoods. They don't need activation, empowerment, more training, financial incentives, or punishments. They don't need to be threatened, called noncompliant, or fired. They need a break. They need care.

Minimally disruptive medicine

Although some of the burden of treatment is not optional, it does not need to be accepted holus bolus. We cannot celebrate progress in alleviating illness and stay mum about the struggles treatment inflicts. Many of these struggles, I believe, are avoidable. Treatment burden does not need to be an immutable aspect of living with disease: the threat of diabetes has nothing to do with the anguish people feel when they are priced out of the technologies (e.g., sugar sensors, insulin pumps) that can alleviate Marge's premeal routines and of the insulins they need to cope, survive, and thrive.

The care patients need, as my colleagues Carl May, Frances Mair, and I wrote in 2009, must be minimally disruptive. This care must focus on advancing the human situation of each patient with the smallest possible healthcare footprint on their lives. It calls for patients and clinicians to shape care to respond well to each patient's situation in a manner designed to fit easily within chaotic lives. This requires drawing from all the relevant and available scientific evidence and from the experience and expertise both parties have.

Minimally disruptive care calls for programs that are easy to access and use, their content coherent, their care continuous and coordinated across all involved. It forbids the delegation of medical errands to patients and families and of considering them as unpaid extensions of healthcare's industrial workforce. Because so much care must be unavoidably completed by the patient, every effort should be made to free self-care from waste by enhancing its meaning, feasibility, and value to the patient. Every portion of work ultimately assigned to the patient must be designed with the most overwhelmed patient in mind.

Consider the routines that evolved as HIV clinics responded to the needs of patients infected with this virus. At a key point in the epidemic, patients went from dying from the HIV infection to living with it thanks to effective, complicated treatments. Patients had to take these treatments consistently — or risk viral resistance and death — as they worked through personal, emotional, psychosocial, and financial difficulties. These clinics understood this. A multidisciplinary team comprised of doctors and nurses, a pharmacist, a social worker, and a receptionist staffed the clinic. As a team, they had to reduce treatment burden, improve treatment adherence, and prevent and attend to complications. The receptionist, for example, would coordinate appointments, facilitate transportation to and from the clinic, verify food and housing, and refill prescriptions. She handed the bag of refilled medicines to patients as they left the clinic after meeting with the team. Working in partnership with patients, many living in impoverished conditions, these clinics successfully controlled the infection in the majority of their patients.

Minimally disruptive care calls for banning noncompliance, because this term and its meaning serve no purpose. Instead, a clearly productive approach diagnoses the patient's situation as reflecting an imbalance between the patient work and the capacity to shoulder it. This diagnosis immediately and intuitively points the way forward and out of the situation: optimize the balance of patient workload to patient capacity.

And optimize is what Ana, a student in our team, did when she took a break to visit her grandmother, Maria Luisa. A Peruvian living with her son and two daughters in Alaska, Maria Luisa lived with multiple chronic conditions requiring a complicated pill regimen. Three days a week she underwent dialysis at a center for three hours in the morning, after which she was so exhausted she had stopped crocheting for her granddaughters. She had been asked to adhere to a boring and bland diet, instead of the colorful Peruvian dishes full of the decadent smells and flavors that she loved. She rarely left the house, her Spanish only useful to communicate with her family and to call friends in Lima.

Ana immediately saw opportunities to implement minimally disruptive care for her grandmother. She organized her medications using a multiday, multidose pillbox. She installed an elevator that allowed Maria Luisa to go between the first and second floors of the house, something she would not do alone during the day for fear of falling down the stairs. She moved dialyses to the afternoon, freeing the mornings for Maria Luisa to restart crocheting. This was a lucky move as two of the dialysis nurses in the afternoon shift spoke Spanish, and this expanded her world. Ana sent the diet restrictions to a dietician in Perú who sent back recipes that were prepared every Sunday for Maria Luisa. Now, she could taste food from her homeland every day without having to cheat, feel guilty, and complicate her medical situation. Expanding her social network, sense of worth and pleasure, and mobilizing some material resources, helped reduce the burden of treatment for Maria Luisa. Palliating her symptoms of fatigue, pain, insomnia, and breathlessness "activated" her; finding success in her self-care and participating in the care of her loved ones "empowered" her.

The work that Ana did is what patient care should do, as most patients and caregivers lack the knowledge, skills, or resources to achieve minimally disruptive care on their own. Her efforts show, however, how kind care that is maximally supportive can reduce the burden of treatment on patients' lives.

Pursuing minimally disruptive care may seem misguided to people who think there is nothing in patients' lives that should take priority over taking care of their own health. In this view, every effort patients can make is warranted to achieve one's health goals. Sometimes that is true, as is often the case under the mortal threat of cancer or the opportunity to receive a lifesaving organ transplant. But for chronic patients without an end in sight such heroics are unwarranted and almost always avoidable. Clinicians must recognize that people (including themselves when they become patients) don't live to be or to become excellent patients. Instead, they draw from patient care the necessary help to gather the health they need to fulfill their obligations to others and to realize their dreams. Thus, some treatments simply will not get implemented, because they don't fit. This may be at odds with those who think that patients should feel fortunate for our excellent care, regardless of how much effort and time it takes to get it. Then, these lucky patients should fulfill their part of the deal and do everything they can to implement the clinician's recommendations. Every clinician who understands their role must have it clear, however, that they are the ones who have the privilege of the bedside, who must be humbled by the possibility to treat each person, to have their trust, to be at their side as they stare ill fate in the eyes.

Patient care must act in the world to reduce violence and promote justice, to respond to anyone and everyone with necessary and safe health care. As I write this, my attention is drawn to the systematic violence against people for their race, ethnicity, nationality, or sexual orientation. Discrimination, isolation, and poverty, unrelenting and unmitigated, screams to their faces that their lives matter less. For those most vulnerable, rendered sick and paralyzed by pervasive and persistent injustice, industrial healthcare responds with its own brand of violence, labeling the person (not the situation) as noncompliant. Patient care, the kind for which we revolt, should be a calm refuge, a safe and just oasis for restoration and regeneration. Patient care must work to reduce the burden it imposes to help people be and do what they must. Rendered minimally disruptive, this care must help every patient live as unhindered as possible by disease and treatment.

Careful and kind care? That is what Marge, Julia, and Maria Luisa want and need to be alive and well.

John

*John is a 55-year-old man. He is overweight. He takes
two different pills daily for diabetes. He also has
hypertension and, until recently, was using a diuretic, a
so-called "water pill." Because he was not meeting the
target for blood pressure control set in the practice's
contract, his doctor added another tablet, a beta
blocker. Now, every time John stands up quickly,
he becomes dizzy. John also has high cholesterol,
depression, a painful lower back, and pain in his feet
from damage to his nerves caused by diabetes.*

*Because of lack of progress in improving any of these
conditions, John's primary care clinician referred him to
the big medical center. Her hope was that he would get
sorted out by a diabetes specialist, by a podiatrist, and
by a dietitian. To attend these appointments, John had
to take time off work and convince his neighbor to give
him a ride. In these visits, the doctors told him that he
needed to avoid salt, fats, and carbs; that he needed
to be active and to exercise despite his painful back
and feet; that he needed to check his feet regularly,*

but John has not been able to see his feet in some time because of his rather large belly.

The doctors repeatedly admonished him for not taking his pills regularly, assuming this must be why he was not making the disease targets … even though he does take them: This is exactly why he gets dizzy when he stands up too quickly. He did not get a chance to contradict them. They also told him to check his blood sugars and to log them. He has been writing down his numbers religiously, bringing them to his appointments. Instead of reviewing the logged numbers, his doctor routinely focuses on a laboratory measure of the average blood sugar levels in the last three months, hemoglobin A1c. In all these encounters, clinicians only discussed John's inability to lower the levels of his A1c, cholesterol, blood pressure, and weight. Not a word about John's difficulties with pain, insomnia, and despair.

Worries about his job keep John up at night. Because of layoffs, John was now the only accountant left of the three the company used to employ. He faced impossible deadlines. To meet these deadlines, he brought work home. He looked hard at the numbers and found problems: the company and his job were in peril. If he were to lose his job, he would also lose his ability to pay his debts, his health insurance premiums, and his mortgage.

But something about home worried him more than paying his mortgage. John's oldest daughter had come back to live with him. When she showed up at the doorstep, she was seeking refuge from an abusive relationship for her and for her two daughters; no escape seemed possible, however, from her addiction to painkillers. John was worried sick about his family.

Slumped in the living room sofa, John reflected about his future, the future of his family, the future of his granddaughters. Dejectedly, he looked at the unopened mail. He noticed the bills and set them aside. He also had a letter from his primary care doctor. He opened it. It was terse. He was not meeting disease control targets. He should look for a new primary care clinician.

There is nothing extraordinary about the story of John. I made him up from the story of many of my patients. I've presented John's story around the world; everywhere, clinicians respond: "Yes, I too know John" and "You just described a large part of my practice." Patients have approached me at the end of my talks with "I am John," "I am Joan," or "You just told the story of my father."

John is an archetype: the patient living in a complicated medical and personal situation that industrial healthcare seems unable to help, yet is ready to shame and blame. It is for patients like him for whom programs to engage, educate, and activate are developed — as if he was in trouble because of ignorance or lack of participation. He is the "inspiration" for insurance schemes that target patients like him with financial penalties to make sure "he has skin in the game." As if the futures of his granddaughters were insufficiently high stakes. He is the scapegoat for poor healthcare outcomes despite escalating healthcare costs.

But John is not the problem. Healthcare needs to care for John, not shame him, or get rid of him. Thinking of John's situation as the problem of healthcare is like blaming the house fire on the smoke escaping through the windows. John is a sign.

A sign.

Like the one depicted in a picture I found online. It showed a tired and soot-covered miner with, allegedly, the last canary used in an

English coal mine. Miners would carry these canaries with them to serve as a signal of the air quality deep inside the mine. As I understand it, if the air were to become toxic, the canaries would become agitated and eventually stop singing. At this point, at the latest, the miners would abandon the mine.

Healthcare became toxic to John. Its responses to John's problems could not and did not improve his situation. His lack of improvement, interpreted as noncompliance, could have been interpreted differently. John, the canary, had stopped singing. But in healthcare, it turns out, that is the canary's fault.

John

Part Two

Elegance

I have spent many proud weekends in a hot and humid place. Surrounded by parents and siblings of eager swimmers, I have cheered my boys on, loudly and in Spanish. This is distinct enough that I have gotten and honored requests to cheer for other kids. Over the years, my "¡vamos, vamos!" has been rewarded with faster times. My boys gained speed by swimming using fewer and more harmonious movements.

As they cruise through the pool, my boys cause just the right amount of turbulence on the pool surface. Improving the efficiency of their moves, eliminating the superfluous and wasteful, has taken years of intense daily practice. They have become elegant swimmers. The energy spent on fighting gravity, resistance, fatigue, pain (some from the bitterly cold water), and other physical and psychological forces is now channeled into just touching the wall first. Their minds, no longer focused on the work of coordination, are on the strategy to swim the race. Their swim caps pulled down over their ears block the sound, but I still cheer. "¡Vamos, vamos!" — and the wall touch, and the arms up, and the fist pump, and the smiles on their faces meeting the sky. They shake hands with the next-lane neighbors and offer a furtive look up to the bleachers. I catch it and take it all in, proud of these most elegant swimmers.

Once you see this in one place, it is everywhere: The elegance of the essential. Effortless masters of their craft, efficiently delegating tasks from consciousness to muscle memory, focusing their energy and attention instead on the next challenge. Careful action now made affordable by the efficient routines executed without waste. The elegance of a thoughtful practice. Taking their time, more deliberate toil than mad rush, to improve their craft.

To care, it seems to me, clinicians must afford deceleration. As a patient, I should feel that what matters to my clinician is going on right now, not tomorrow, not with the next patient, or with the one that left earlier. This time together with me needs to be slowed down, thin-sliced, and understood. In the depth of our encounter, we must think through, work through, feel through, and talk through my problems as a patient. These moments generate whatever will follow: more testing, gathering other opinions, considering other forms of care, waiting it out, treatment. We will slow time down, not to simply lengthen it, but to look deep into the situation. And to look again. To inspect and to respect. Without investing in this time together, misunderstanding and missteps will follow. Walk carefully to avoid tripping. To care, patient care must decelerate and deepen.

Yet, healthcare is focused on improving its efficiency, not to make care more elegant, but to simply do more with less. A strong emphasis on efficiency has convinced many of my colleagues that the unhurried consultation is a relic, no longer an ingredient in the intelligent design of how healthcare companies deliver healthcare. Indeed, the unhurried consultation, between patients, their families, and a competent, careful, and kind clinician, looks very inefficient. It is true that medicine has accumulated many useless rituals that persist despite their low value. Putting a stethoscope on the neck and over the carotid artery to listen for bruits, for example. It is just not accurate enough to detect or rule out blockages that can cause strokes. On the other hand, some rituals — the words, the gestures, the touch — can demonstrate care and foster trust. In the hands of experienced clinicians, listening, examining, counseling, and listening again — a string of smoothly concatenated actions and purposeful inactions — will quickly follow one another without waste and seem unhurried to the patient. Caring is not meant to be efficient, it is meant to be elegant.

Against a timer, clinicians in charge of the choreography of the encounter may decide to cut the dance short. They may skip some moves, some of them important. They will ask yes/no questions, interrupt patients' answers within 11 seconds, narrowly focus or completely omit the exam, and offer one or two "next steps" before holding the doorknob and motioning the end of the visit. Engaging patients to understand what matters to them, offering explanation, and working to weave treatment into their routines — these elegancies and kindnesses will fade, displaced by tasks that clinicians must complete, such as documentation (for billing) and billing. Analysis and reflection about *this patient* replaced for convenience with the semi-automatic application of algorithms for *patients like this*. Discussion with wise colleagues replaced with the next visit. Any vestige of elegant practice interrupted by urgencies without importance, by cybernetic demands the computer on the physician's desk makes for more data. In these ways, the efficiencies gained do not make healthcare elegant because they interfere with care. It is fast, but not better, with extraneous movements that disrupt, interrupt, and corrupt clinical encounters.

In medicine, time imposes a certain oppression. The oppressor, of course, is not the clock, but the invisible hand that sets the duration of the visit to an arbitrarily brief time. In the last 20 years, encounters have gotten busier. The pressure for clinicians to see more patients in less time blocks other worthwhile actions: calling patients back, discussing puzzling features of a patient presentation with other clinicians, keeping up-to-date with medical knowledge, or reflecting or reading about a misstep or a bad outcome. Clinicians must also take time to take care of their own well-being. These essentials are delegated to others, to later, or to never. That the apparent efficiencies gained by overclocking the doctor will later create waste escapes scrutiny. That a patient's situation was wrongly appreciated and now requires review in a new visit may in fact be valued favorably when contracts pay doctors and healthcare companies per visit. If the patient situation has now worsened, this may require more aggressive or specialized testing and treatment. The push for more and briefer visits may result in efficiency without effectiveness. It may pass for healthcare, but it is not patient care.

This inelegance has been obvious to many patients and clinicians in underserved systems. The system, understaffed and underfunded, is really kept afloat by the personal sacrifice of its staff and the generosity of the patients who gratefully tolerate the limited service available. Speed and disrespect in these systems are a constant threat to human dignity.

Conversely, when resources are available, bloated administration, poor organization of services, profiteering, and corruption waste those resources. In some countries, the ideological battle over universal access through a publicly funded system can manifest as marked reductions in funding that "demonstrate" the inadequacy of the public system — appointments get shorter, waiting lists longer. Where the invisible hand of the market controls healthcare, it is the extraction of excessive profits from the system by investors that starves it of the resources it needs to support careful and kind patient care. Abusive profiteering in underfunded systems tattoos a new high-water mark of exploitation on the frustrated faces of patients, particularly patients least able to complain, negotiate hurdles, or garner special favors. When resources are tight, because of scarcity, incompetence, politics, or profit seeking, people in Hubert Humphrey's "shadows of life," the sickest and humblest, may get healthcare, but not the kind that cares for and about them.

The pressures and interruptions of fast medicine can make any clinician seem inexpert, substituting her expertise in elegant practice for an ersatz expertise in processing patients. I get many calls from patients, often family and friends, who need a second opinion. Invariably, the situation is complicated. But it is also common to see people in whom the powerful, expensive, and harmful tools of medicine have been used too much and too soon. The opposite is also common: people, often of limited means, are in trouble because those tools were used too little or too late. These people are in trouble because healthcare was rushed and careless. Because providing healthcare did not mean receiving patient care.

Perhaps this threat is not new. Raymond Pruitt, a physician, joined Mayo Clinic in the 1940s, later started Mayo Medical School, and became its first dean. A few years after completing his tenure as dean, Pruitt gave an important speech to his colleagues. In it, he reminisced about the Mayo Clinic he met on arrival decades before. Doctors had time, he noted, to have unhurried consultations, to review tough cases with colleagues, to have the conversations that support friendships, to reflect and, usually at the end of the week, to capture what was learned and what was to be learned. Many did research on Fridays as their patients journeyed home.

He noticed the changes he had observed: how Mayo Clinic had become known as a cost-containment champion. He worried that in doing so, the institution may have advanced its economic margin but put at risk what he called "the margin of elegance." Pruitt had seen the deliberate elegance of Mayo Clinic — the doctors who worked together, walking, never running, with the patient who was carefully inspected and kindly respected — and was worried it would get lost under the disciplines of the administration. The year: 1977.

Forty years later, elegance can still be found, but one must explore the margins of healthcare for it. This is what my colleagues from the Center for Innovation at Mayo decided to do in 2010. They compiled moments of "deep human connection" in the hospital.

> As the attending physician and the other trainees moved on to the next case, an intern took a second look and noticed the patient was upset. He stayed behind and sat calmly at the bedside.
>
> The patient's daughter had just arrived from out of state late in the afternoon and had missed meeting with the surgeon. Later that night, in the quiet of the hospital night shift, the surgeon stopped by on his way home. "He was in his street clothes," she remembered.

Nothing heroic, nothing extravagant. Just plain care rendered extraordinary by the pressures of a high-value healthcare that sees small kindnesses as a luxury.

The push for more with less has not only affected the experience of receiving care but has spilled onto the experience of living with disease. Healthcare has shifted work from the healthcare professionals to less expensive technicians capable only of partial work and onto patients and their families. Managers speak of teamwork and attribute the magical property of "keeping everyone on the same page" to the electronic medical record and other technologies. But the to-do list on that page assigns increasingly more tasks to the patient team. They must do the work and pay the price. Patients must negotiate with administrative personnel to access their own records, ensure these are shared across systems with incompatible electronic systems, and comprehend incomprehensible and often incorrect bills. They must promote communication and coordination between doctors to ensure their recommendations are consistent and safe when implemented together. They must discover who should be contacted to address a new concern or to verify and correct a prescription, bill, test requisition, or record. Healthcare continually thwarts any hope of making illness and treatment elegant parts of a person's life.

Sometimes the quest for efficiency in the healthcare system also reduces waste for the patient. An efficient clinic that stays on time means less wait time for the patient. Placing services that patients usually use together close to each other may improve communication among them and reduce travel time for the patient. Some healthcare companies, ThedaCare in Wisconsin and Virginia Mason in Washington, for example, have championed these efficiencies using the Lean approach adapted from the Toyota Production System. A careful review of their approach, however, shows its limitation: it stops at the clinic door. Reducing waste for the patient in their self-care at home or at work is not on their process maps. Thus, when efficiency benefits the patient, it is more often the result of a happy coincidence than of a disciplined adherence of healthcare company managers to patient-centeredness.

Bonnie is a writer and travels for work. She is also a mother of two and a person with type 1 diabetes. An expert patient, she has almost three decades of experience with this condition. Traveling, however, with its changing rules, inconsistent security routines from one airport to the other, time zone crossings, unpredictable opportunities to eat, bursts of running to make connections, and crammed spaces — the middle seat, the bathroom — offer all the challenges an elegant patient may love to avoid. Bonnie, however, loves to travel.

Her work, like her family, is central to her personal realization. She arrived earlier than necessary to the security screening. She pulled out the extra insulin pump from her carry-on (to avoid the X-ray machine) and alerted the agent that she had another one and a continuous glucose monitor sensor both connected to her body. To avoid the scanners, which can ruin the pumps, she asked for a pat-down. Her machines and hands were checked for explosives. She smiled, waiting to respond to the unexpected. Later, at 38,000 feet, in the midst of flight-attendants-must-sit-down turbulence, her blood sugars became stubbornly high; the connection between her insulin pump and the skin behind her right arm needed change. In the crammed space of 38A, with her scarf cleverly deployed as a privacy screen, she moved precisely and quickly, around her clothing, on a violently shaking plane, and changed her connector. Through this, she would have appeared calm, determined, and in control. Her glorious smile the exclamation point of having put herself together. Of getting better sugar readings. Of coming home safely to her family. Of doing it all over again the next time.

Because treatments for diabetes, high blood pressure, depression, and other chronic conditions are lifelong, they must be woven into life, interlacing threads with the warps of family, friends, labor, recreation, and community. This weaving, like the art of the skilled workers of the Andes, must be planned yet flexible, and must realize the themes that run through the length of the tapestry. The weaving must account for accents and deviations and must respond to new challenges and opportunities the artisan may or may not have imagined.

Patients with chronic disease must become masters of self-care; they must learn to operate at two speeds. The hands move the loom and threads quickly and precisely, their work economical and efficient, without wasted turns or unnecessary steps. The patterns on the cloth, however, only emerge after many hours or days of work. The connection between each weft and the whole tapestry is difficult to glean if one looks only briefly or is drawn only to the hands. Over time, the quality and meaning of the work emerges. The artisan appears patient, unhurried, elegant. An elegance born of wasting no energy, time, or attention. The elegance of taking no shortcuts, of being careful, of respect. Of stopping to review, to undo and restart if necessary.

The work of being a patient can be a fulfilling part of a person's life. There are the small triumphs of figuring out how to get through the day without being stumped by fatigue or pain, of improvising in the routine of surprises, of seeming spontaneous thanks to meticulous planning, of kicking uncertainty and disease in the ass!

Doing this well can redefine health when disease cannot be cured. It is hard work made harder or easier by how healthcare organizations foster moments of "deep human connection." By their choice to walk and not run. By their commitment to bring elegance in from the margins, even at the expense of the economic margin. By their ability to draw patients and clinicians to unhurriedly create treatment programs that sensibly and feasibly address the patient situation. Without waste or rush, care must be elegant.

Solidarity

Mark Linzer is the physician leader of general medicine at Hennepin County Medical Center. This is a county-run safety net health system, designed to meet the needs of the sick regardless of socioeconomic fortune. Upon arriving at Hennepin, he found a chaotic clinic, a joyless mess, its walls lined with faded signs and Post-It notes. Patients sat restless, seeking relief through the fog of their language barriers, the effect of pain killers, and the sickening worry that the streets of Minneapolis will sooner or later end their lives. Despair had taken hold of the spirit of the nurses and clinicians, painting their faces with hurried indifference. On busier days, the staff saw those in the waiting room with trepidation, as if they were organizing an occupying army, mounting a siege, and plotting an overwhelming attack. Just a few months before, these clinicians had joined the clinic, motivated to serve the dispossessed; now, they were burned out and ready to quit. Administrators figured that the clinic was not only chaotic but also inefficient. Their models indicated that clinicians could care for far more people. Mark's own analysis demonstrated that these clinicians went home to spend hours completing documentation and billing tasks. Depleted, these clinicians could not give more attention, care, or love to more patients. Mark noticed.

And then Mark bucked the trend. He slowed down the pace. He stabilized the teams. He lengthened patient visits. He cleaned up and decluttered the walls. He simplified policies and helped managers see the time clinicians were spending caring for patients. He reduced the waste caused by confusion, distrust, and noise.

And then he did some more. He went under the bridges. There, he found and talked directly with the people his clinic was hoping to serve. He didn't seek to interpret their words or to bring the "voice of the customer" to the clinic; rather, he gave voice to these marginalized people — as if someone had armed them with a megaphone — taking them from *they* to *us*. From alien to kindred. He took his guitar and raised funds in the local pub to support their care. He cared for people, those doing the caring and those seeking care. People began to smile a little more. Professionals talked with each other and supported each other a bit more often. The waiting room remained full, but the patients' wait was now hopeful, *they* now *we*, rooting for *our* success. Everyone noticed.

Unlike Mark, industrial healthcare often fails to notice the people at the frontlines of care. Being noticed — by investors, ranking makers, the press — takes a higher priority for these companies. The brochures rarely highlight their ability to care: their capacity for elegant unhurried care where patients are not a blur; in which clinicians and patients collaborate and partner; and in which the care is scientific, regenerative, and highly personal. Patients, in the ads and the carefully manicured public relations stories, are the objects of the industry's prowess, their "human interest" merely a prop. Industrial healthcare sees them as a means to their corporate end.

Not Mark. Dr. Linzer noticed the people who were there to care for patients and took their side. Of course, sides had not been formally drawn yet. These professionals were not fully aware that their sense of medicine, nursing, and patient care was at odds with the goals and methods of industrial healthcare. But they knew their daily work increasingly involved overcoming their own demoralization and siding with their patients. Mark joined the staff in their struggle, his struggle, the struggle. In his own way, Mark demonstrated the antithesis of greed.

Mark had the education, the experience, and the position to feel responsible for those less fortunate. He could be influential on behalf of the weak. And he made choices that offered him benefits, not materially but humanly. He moved the clinic forward, not by threatening loss of income or by promising a greater share in the profits. He reminded clinicians of their calling, casting a shared vision of careful and kind care. He showed them how each patient is a suffering comrade, and his team noticed. They rejected casting patients as *them*, as a mountain of work, as an enemy besieging the clinic, as a customer who is always right, as human ATMs. Instead they relearned to see one of their own in every one of them. In doing so, Dr. Linzer and his team made a huge discovery, one that will not be printed on glossy corporate or academic pages. The solution is not in moderating greed. It is in solidarity.

Solidarity is a stubborn human trait. Stubborn as are the demons that compel gangs of humans to devalue, subjugate, abuse, and destroy others. Amidst the horrors we cause, our better selves improbably figure out how to care for each other.

It took the March of Dimes, the massive humble contribution of millions, to fund the development of the Salk polio vaccine. When it became available, it was offered for free to the pharmaceutical industry for its manufacturing and distribution. The World Health Organization, UNICEF, the U.S. Centers for Disease Control, the

Gates Foundation, the Rotary Club, and others collaborated to erad-
icate polio from the planet. As I write this, the world is on the verge
of declaring polio, including the infantile paralysis and suffering
accompanying it, all but gone. This success did not stem from profit
seeking, competition, or promotion of individual responsibility. It
could not. Solidarity fueled the polio eradication effort. In 2016,
an article in *Forbes* magazine missed the point by asking how much
money Salk had forfeited by not patenting the vaccine. The world
did not miss the point. Humanity is poised to do this again, developing what appears to be an effective vaccine for the Ebola virus, erad-
icating it from Liberia and other West African countries.

A healthcare company, noticing the problem of access Dr. Linzer's
patients faced, could ask how might we ensure access for patients that
better support our bottom line? Instead, solidarity calls for a different
question: How might we co-create with patients and communities
the best ways to use our limited resources? Co-creation of this vision
with patients is tough. Leaders, on boards and in executive offices,
will need to pay special attention to patients who have less visibility,
a muted voice, or face complex circumstances. *They* must be noticed
and their plight must be ours.

The big bucks are paid to creative, insightful, and decisive executives who are tasked with making healthcare sustainable and innovative. It is neither creative nor insightful to eliminate less profitable
services and exclude or wait-list patients whose care hurts economic
performance. The decision to exclude may seem easy to make for
those judging performance through the optics of greed, but this is
no longer our lens. Because every time one of us is excluded, we have
a problem.

Compassion is not enough to guide decision-making in patient
care. Industrial healthcare leaders can probably claim sympathy
for patients. But the sufferers remain safely *other*, and this distance

allows leaders to make "tough" decisions; any pain caused finds fault elsewhere, sometimes even with the sufferer. "The patient did not file the correct form on time." "Why couldn't she just follow our protocols?" "It was her job, her only job, to come to the appointment." These are real statements hurled at a low-literacy woman who, with great dignity, cared for her disabled son and elderly mother, paying her bills by holding two low-paying jobs. I cared for her knowing that when she came to our appointments, I would see a huge smile, a winning and contagious one despite missing several teeth. On a good day, we connected. Her struggle felt like our struggle. Her tears, our tears. No distance. Through conversation, we ended up sharing points of view, analyses, and outlooks. The tough way forward covered by walking together in her shoes. Empathy became solidarity. And solidarity smiled.

Smiles are Sree Koka's business. As a prosthodontist, he replaces missing teeth with tooth prostheses, to help people eat, speak, and smile. When Sree was completing an executive MBA, the students were asked to present about the meaning they found in their work. Sree's soft discourse, unassuming, quietly let the before-after pictures do the talking. Each miraculously full smile was a testimony to artisanship, teamwork, and trust, the glorious end to a long treatment. Although Sree's peers at the MIT MBA were quite successful, they responded to his presentation with sweet envy, seeing real meaning in his work.

Sree moved to the West Coast armed with a glistening MBA and opened a new dental practice that focused on patients supported by the generous California Medicaid program. One by one, through word of mouth, patients heard of Dr. Koka and his practice, the only prosthodontist in San Diego receiving Medicaid-covered patients. After care, patients returned to the practice, but not to show off their smile or tell stories of better nutrition or speech. Rather, a man thanked the dentist for not judging him when he first came with teeth rotten from drug addiction. A woman wanted the good doctor to know that after 15 years she had gathered the courage to apply for a job; she screamed from the threshold of the practice door, "I am back in the world!" Sree showed me her picture, covering her mouth from the before and the after images. The eyes, not the teeth, told the story. Sree smiled as I discovered how her eyes had acquired a happy confidence. Patient and doctor, satisfied together, proud of each other.

Dr. Koka's practice is facing the financial struggles of a startup, but its professionals have pledged to be successful by prioritizing care, by eschewing unnecessary nice-to-get tests or treatments that are standard elsewhere, and by making their own prostheses when they can. They aim to pay themselves a good-enough salary, about the median salary for dentists in the U.S. Fundamentally, they budget empathic care for anyone that comes calling.

Mark and Sree, by education, position, and personal virtue, noticed. They noticed the situation of their patients. They noticed the conditions of their lives. They noticed the situation of the practice, its practitioners, and their capacity to respond to patient needs. Their deliberate approach — to prioritize care and subordinate money as simply a means to that end — is revolutionary enough. Their commitment to serve the silenced and the marginalized divorces them from industrial healthcare. We must, as they did, care for those kept alien, celebrate the mattering of their lives, and make addressing their struggle our struggle. Our revolution, fueled by solidarity, must abolish banal indifference, unintentional cruelty, and careless greed. Our patient revolution must leave out no one. No healthcare refugees. No second-class citizens. All lives worthy. All smiles precious.

Love

Dear Doctor,

Something happened in February. Since then, the signals were clear: It is all about money. I could tell because of the difficulties getting appointments, tests, and referrals. The appointment reminder letters were fine, but not the stuff about how I should prefer to follow up not with you, my specialist, but with my primary care doctor.

I turned 65 in February. That birthday made me suspicious of every decision we took together. Was this for my benefit or was this to reflect the directive you got to discourage visits with "Medicare patients?" I hate that label, as if Medicare was a disease. Turning 65 made me a healthcare undesirable. The healthcare company had not figured out how to make money when caring for patients for whom Medicare pays the bills. I am one of them. I ruined your practice's "payer mix." I should back off and find another healthcare company. Break up with you. Go look for another doctor.

But I love you. Some politicians, in pushing reform, insist that people should be able to keep their doctor. I think they know that some people love their doctors. Love? It is not my dependence on you, your skills, or the doors to healthcare that you open for me. It is not being in love with you, entering some Freudian transference by which I cannot live without you.

It is that I love you. I find you not just capable, but that you see me. That you see me in my world and witness my struggle through it. That you listen without judgment. That you imagine your care playing out in the drama of my life, not in the simplified version of it that other doctors I have seen imagine and your "best practices" assume. This is not professional politeness or rehearsed communication. It is you, Doctor, loving me back. Expressing concern and distress when things don't work out. Mobilizing your expertise to come up with another approach for my situation, one that will fit me. After things changed, after February, I noticed you just did not go along. You discreetly showed your repudiation of the business letters, of the "money first" signals that sought to corrupt our communion and reduce it to a transaction. I particularly appreciated your promise to see me no matter what, Medicare and all.

I must admit, in my cynicism, that I suspected your promises empty, until you gave me your cellphone number and offered to pick it up anytime. Thank you for loving me back.

Your patient.

Maybe.

I have been a diabetes doctor for 10 years and a clinician working in the privilege of the bedside for 20. In all that time, I have not had any patient say I love you.

Type 2 diabetes is a chronic condition that is often devoid of symptoms. I don't operate, rarely alleviate, and almost never cure. In contrast with my colleagues across the hall who cure hyperthyroidism and tumors of the pituitary gland, I get no Christmas gifts or cards from patients. Our routine is don't overeat, move more, take your meds, and see you next year. Because next year you will still have diabetes. Perhaps love needs drama and tragedy, and these are increasingly rare, thankfully, in my practice. So, no love for Dr. Montori.

Maybe.

I have felt, a million times, my patients' respect, their concern for my own well-being, and their humor. The paradox: They came for care, yet often started our encounters by asking about me and my loved ones. How is your father? Are the kids still swimming? You look tired. Are you getting enough rest? Not polite small talk. Rarely about the weather, a major feat in the climate smorgasbord of Minnesota. They came for care, but their opening gambit was an unhurried expression of care. Their questions tell me that they listened to my answers and retained them in the three- or six-month interval since their last visit. These are sick people participating in constrained visits; yet they opt to invest precious time in caring for and about me. They are quick to forgive my lapses and my delays. They listen patiently to my stories. It is as if they love me, their doctor.

Maybe.

My patients don't know that there are many days in which I would rather not see them. It may be because I have other things I do that are often exhilarating and interesting. Work with my research team is often fun, challenging, and important. My patients don't know that on days when I am reluctant to see them I feel sluggish, like I'm running in thigh-deep mud. I feel guilty, privileged, and humbled when I notice the zip codes. Five, seven, even 10 hours of driving and their only appointment is with me. It is on these days that they win me over. They pry open my soul and we see each other: When it is harder for me, it is easier for me to see how hard each day must be for them. We connect.

Wrapped in this love, we understand, solve problems, laugh a lot — and we cry quite a bit too. That these emotions emerge and that the visits take longer stresses my trainees. They choose endocrinology because it involves the careful understanding of the elegant mechanisms governing hormone levels and the objective numbers that represent them. No crying over an elevated HbA1c level! Biology offers an illusion of straightforwardness that fades with every patient, unable to sufficiently represent each patient's situation. Somehow, trainees don't learn this; the illusion persists and it shapes how they care. When care is wrapped in love, however, crying happens. The patients and I know that these loving relationships help to recover from a setback, to regain perspective or hope, and to reframe a goal with compassion and self-forgiveness. We know that love heals.

At the end of these days in which I reluctantly participate, I frequently feel energized. I get back home with stories to share. I feel loved and, maybe, my patients feel that I love them back.

In my research, I have watched hundreds of videos of clinical encounters. They show patients and clinicians in primary care and specialty care, in the hospital, and in emergency rooms. These videos have shown me that my experience is neither unique nor routine. Not many of my colleagues or their patients laugh or cry in the encounters we have taped, but some do. They laugh about themselves, a quick joke to lighten the mood or to avoid crying. Their visits resemble a sweet human dance: the air between them filled with invisible connections, made and dissolved in the trial and error of learning to be together and to care for and about each other.

The magic and love that empower the sick and miraculously nourish the healer are alive and well, but at risk of extinction. They are crowded out by the forces of efficiency, fighting to emerge between the technique and jargon of clinical transactions. "How can I help you?" The patient begins. Eleven seconds later, the clinician's silent body language interrupts. Eyes on the computer, the doctor types. Is the patient allowed to interrupt? The doctor questions and expects brief answers. More typing. Eyes have lost contact. The patient gambles to reconnect, but the clinician misses the hint. "I see," he says. He performs a focused exam and lists next steps. "The receptionist at the desk will help you make a return appointment. Any questions?" 3, 2, 1. "OK, then. Feel free to contact my nurse if you have concerns. Please fill out the patient satisfaction survey."

These videos show clinicians and patients awkwardly struggling to love. Failure of love to prevail has consequences. Clinicians may be less able to understand the patient's situation, to see the patient in high definition. Without love, the patient with very high blood sugar levels will not disclose that she lost her job and has not been able to afford her diabetes medications. Without this possibly embarrassing disclosure, the clinician will misdiagnose the problem as uncontrolled diabetes and offer more intensive and expensive treatment. Without time to muster the courage to ask, clarify, or correct, the patient will go home with another prescription, another frustration. With complains unresolved, she must seek care elsewhere.

These same clinicians may find it hard to see the value of their care; they get through the day carrying out meaningless administrative tasks that crowd out care, doing more but never enough, and stressing under the unreasonable burdens of giving perfect and efficient care. Almost half of U.S. physicians work while exhausted, depleted, or unable to care. When clinicians feel burned out, they are more likely to cut back on patient time, seek other occupations, and leave medical practice.

Clinicians and patients quickly learn that time is of the essence, that the discussion must be to the point, and that there are questions and concerns that may have to wait. Documentation and payer-incentivized care bring in money, laughing and crying do not. They learn to make the best of these transactional visits, as efficiency pressures fill the space between them, preventing them from forming new and enduring connections.

How is your father? Are the kids still swimming? You look tired. Are you getting enough rest? Her doctor asks, remembering his patient's worries from three months ago. The patient loves that her doctor remembers. She feels heard, seen. Invisible connections are formed, others strengthened. She was not sure if she should tell her doctor this, but she is struggling with her oldest son. The doctor leans forward. She lowers her gaze and her voice. He touches her hand. Love, not time, is of the essence. Her son is in trouble. Perhaps her sugars are high because she is worried sick. "Go on." Her doctor listens, cares, loves.

Maybe.

Amanda

Twenties. Me too. Very thin. Poor. Alone. Terminal from a curable infection. Her lungs destroyed by indifference, poverty, and tuberculosis. I don't remember the exact time, but there was no one else in the ward. The end of the afternoon? Under very tall ceilings, the sun's rays disinfected the long room. She lay breathing in the last of the 15 beds.

No mask for me. This too we had in common: the system showed no love for her or for me, leaving me vulnerable to the germ that was killing her. Oh well. I was Superman, well-nourished and immortal.

No one else around. Shortness of breath. A little oxygen through the nose had not been sufficient. Earlier, we had built a mask with a plastic bottle: two holes covered by little bits of latex glove. This helped her breathe easier, but not as well as she would have on morphine or sedatives, which we did not have. Peace only came from the amber bathing of the sun setting in the unit. Silence.

I don't remember her name.

I don't remember having much else to do for her. There was no one else in the unit, except for 15 patients at different stages of desperation. Amanda, let's call her Amanda, was the most desperate. Alone. Short of breath.

I reached for her left hand, and she held mine. Her eyes turned to my eyes. I didn't know what else to do.

(Don't sit on the patient's bed ...)

(Fuck it!)

I sat facing her. Holding her left hand. A tear or two on her face. I had nothing to offer. Her right arm lifted in my direction, and her body pivoted to the left. She was moving toward me. I turned around and sat at her side. My arm slid behind her back. I held her closer as she sat up a bit.

(She will breathe better ... I hope).

She was barely breathing. She was dying in my arms for lack of justice.

I told her stories, I think. I said something, but perhaps no words came out. Her eyes said something too, but, tired, they closed. I closed my eyes too, I guess. I knew. I think she knew too, calmly.

She was dying in my arms.

I am now holding her tight. My breathing following hers, like his steps in sync with hers when an old couple takes a long, intimate walk. Her eyes opened one last time. She is too young to stop. Too young to stop. I felt her go. Leave. Death. Not alone.

Did she feel love?

I pulled myself from under her thin torso, making sure her head softly

touched the pillow beneath. I covered this injustice with unjustifi-
ably white sheets. I stood alone. Unaware of the other patients who
had watched, those who could, respectfully from their beds.

The older woman in the next bed, the 14th one, outstretched her
right hand toward me and met my gaze with a reassuring smile. She
held my hand between hers, soothing my rage. I sat by her and we
cried, briefly, together. I don't remember her name.

Integrity

In 1991, Gordon Guyatt, a Canadian physician, took charge of training internal medicine doctors at McMaster University. As he began his tenure, he made two key decisions. The first one was to promote the teaching and learning of evidence-based medicine. Evidence-based medicine taught trainees that medical decisions had to consider the best available research evidence. This simple and now obvious idea transformed medical education and research, and changed patient care worldwide.

Secondly, Guyatt decided to prohibit pharmaceutical representatives from interacting with trainees. To him, the pharmaceutical industry was successfully peddling products, not education. At the time, these two decisions were very controversial and cost Guyatt the support and friendship of many colleagues. However, they were coherent, requiring that patients be cared for based on science, not on meals and road trips with attractive salespeople. Guyatt's trainees experienced medical education without the contradictions of science and money, and through his decisions, they could appreciate and learn the value of his integrity.

In 2002, drawn by his pioneering work, I started a two-year training program under Dr. Guyatt's mentorship. When I returned to Mayo Clinic, I started a research program in evidence-based medicine, the Knowledge and Encounter Research (KER) Unit. At first, I made plans to seek funding from charitable foundations, government agencies, and corporations. Our parent organization, Mayo Clinic, encourages partnerships with healthcare corporations and their research and development programs. To protect the science, the scientists, and the institution, it has stringent rules to manage potential conflicts of interest. With these encouragements and protections, we could take funding from for-profit corporations, but should we?

The work of the KER Unit is intended to help clinicians and patients make health and care decisions. Research has repeatedly shown that corporate funding is strongly associated with research results favoring the sponsor. Because of how money can influence doctors — and everyone else — corporations generously fund researchers, institutions, clinicians who are opinion leaders, and patient advocacy groups. Naively, researchers dedicated to the pursuit of discovery and clarity often assume they and their science are above the influence of money. The mere presence of corporate funds, however, could offer another explanation for our research findings and for the recommendations we make now and in the future, even if (we think) money had had no influence on us or our work.

Integral to our commitment to make patient care better through research was the unit's decision to prioritize the trustworthiness of our work. In defense of this integrity, the KER Unit investigators decided to never accept funding from for-profit corporations. The result is that our unit's independence has enabled us to investigate and denounce the corrupting effect of corporate funding on research and clinical care. This policy also adds coherence to our

work, discourse, and academic lives. As with everything that is difficult to do, yet worth doing, our commitment to integrity in the way
we fund and conduct research is a source of identity and pride for us.

Here, we must discuss incoherence of professional values and actions,
contradictions between mission and policies, and trust-busting
alternative explanations. Loss of integrity may be the original sin
that ended up corrupting healthcare away from its fundamental mission of caring. Loss of integrity — along with incoherence and contradictions — abounds in industrial healthcare. Leaders must work
hard to stand at the pivot of a seesaw, harmonizing conflicting goals,
finding congruence between them. Instead, they often jump off the
seesaw, giving up on what is *ideal*, hoping that *expeditious* will do.
When *expeditious* rules, however, it finds *ideal* too expensive, imprac-
tical, unsuitable to meet the challenges of a changing healthcare
landscape. We must adapt, *expeditious* says, compromising until we
can no longer recognize ourselves or remember why we went into
patient care. Those reasons are left gathering dust in a book about
ideal. The unintended consequence is the erosion of a sense of coherence between the context of care and the care itself.

Incoherence and insults to integrity are devastating to frontline
patient care professionals — and those who must trust them to get
better. I am convinced that these contribute significantly to clinician disaffection, and frustration with and abandonment of clinical
practice. "Delivering" care incessantly, continuously, and instantaneously, while simultaneously attending to the demands of documentation and billing, is soul-crushing. So is the system that
allocates half the time of an encounter to satisfy those administrative demands. This system leaves too little time to understand the
situation of each patient, to order only the necessary tests, and to
consider carefully what aspect of the patient's situation demands
action and what action the situation demands. Instead, we order

tests and treatments according to what is recommended for people *like our patient* and what is necessary to meet publicly reported standards of quality and to collect income bonuses for ourselves. This creates an insidious sense of corruption in the mission: lots of healthcare, little care.

Patients understand that their clinicians are now subject to pressures to increase demand for the use of expensive tools and services — the new surgeon (be it the robot or its glamorous operator), the new imaging machine, or the new wing of the hospital. "Ask your doctor if you need this service," says the Choosing Wisely campaign, urging patients to play defense and avoid unnecessary tests and treatments instead of placing their trust in the integrity of their clinicians. Loss of trust — in the competence of clinicians and in the reasons for clinicians' recommendations — reduces the efficacy of their interventions, including the well-being that comes with truly being cared for, and adds to patient work spent in obtaining second opinions or pursuing legal or administrative actions.

Low-integrity healthcare pitches the autonomy of the consumer against the integrity of the clinician. Patients, buying into the idea that they are consumers in a marketplace in which you must "ask your doctor about," show up demanding care that they don't need. Fulfilling these requests, reinforced by financial rewards linked to satisfaction surveys, offends clinicians' sense of what is right for the patient and interferes with the careful design of care with and for this patient, not for the one in the commercial.

Low-integrity healthcare pitches the entrepreneurship of the clinician against the vulnerability of the patient. Advertisements and referrals for tests, procedures, and treatments of unknown or unclear value to secure profits connect clinical practice to the dark ages of the snake oil salesman. This includes the oncologist who "won't give up" while he profits from infusing one more round of chemotherapy in his clinic, the surgeon who offers to robotically remove the uterus of an asymptomatic woman, and the cardiology van in which patients indiscriminately receive a carotid ultrasound and a referral for "full evaluation" at the new vascular center. The undervaluation of healthcare integrity squanders trust and reduces the sense of worth of the people in healthcare, their institutions, and the value of what they do together. It deforms the congruent practice of patient care: at best, it renders care incoherent; at worst, all sense of care vanishes.

As we stand tall at the pivot of the seesaw, integrity helps us figure out how to leverage the practical to elevate the important, how to resist the forces that compel us to jump, to give up, and to comply. On reflection, I think I learned about this very early in my life, at home. My father's life changed dramatically in July 1980. Democracy had returned to Perú after 12 years of military rule. The newly elected president had asked my father to abandon his private life and preside over the national oil company. My father accepted the challenge, but seemed to age overnight. International oil operators and consultants wanted to secure lucrative contracts. Politicians pressured my father to place their family members in the company's employment. Supervisors and employees, without a sense of purpose or accomplishment, passively sabotaged any reforms.

That year, as Christmas approached, the base of our tree began to disappear behind piles of very large gifts. Many of these were cardboard boxes without any wrapping, with a business card attached. Some contained original art and some expensive imported liquor. A large wooden trunk with my dad's name engraved on the side was also delivered — it too was filled with exclusive bottles. I was fascinated with these gifts, my eyes wide with expectation. Not my dad. He would arrive late at night, walk by the tree, and agree with my mother to send all the gifts back. "They are trying to buy me."

Two years later, he was out of the job. His unilateral exercise to pre-serve his own integrity and that of the company, by resisting the allure of gifts, incentives, and the asphyxiating pressures from pow-erful quarters, cost him most of his "friends" and, thanks to corrupt political and judiciary processes, his freedom. Treachery and prison caused him to suffer tremendously, but he never had any regrets. I came to learn over the years that this is who he was — his actions, his practices, his convictions and principles all one. His integrity endures, meaningfully mattering decades later, and is my standard.

If the experiences of my father or of Gordon Guyatt are typical, acting with integrity in contradiction to industrial healthcare will be urgent, painful, lonely, and rewarding. The patient revolution must work hard to foster the protection and promotion of personal and institutional integrity. Integrity is the gravitational force that holds people true while they care for patients, who in turn respond with trust, if not love. We must chip away at the structural and operational insults to the integrity of people, furthering, through open dialogue, a sense of what is fundamentally true about care. We must promote coherent work and trust in each other. In pursuing integrity, the revolution will find a common and universal point of reference from which to foster patient care without contradictions.

Part Three

Timelessness

Minutes spent at the bedside with a dying patient and her family.

Minutes completing the billing record.

Minutes learning about a patient's clandestine insulin injections at work because the boss objects to the use of needles.

Minutes completing required physician training designed to improve patient satisfaction scores.

Minutes listening quietly to a patient mourning the loss of her oldest son, missing his smile, tormented by doubt and guilt.

Minutes in which clinicians discuss difficult cases and difficult feelings with colleagues.

Minutes that clinicians set aside to reflect, read, and research.

Silent minutes to listen to patients, minutes to co-create carefully their treatment plans.

Elegant and unhurried minutes.

Minutes of meaningful care in which time stops and grows deeper and thicker.

When time is money, these minutes are all the same, or worse, minutes that make money matter more and crowd out the other minutes. As profitable minutes take priority, the depletion of those other minutes, the richest ones, the ones that matter to both patients and doctors, impoverishes care. Because of how healthcare companies make money, of how they get paid to "deliver healthcare," it matters to their bottom line how time is spent. Their focus on value — the contemporary incarnation of efficiency, how much of a desirable outcome can be obtained from each unit of resource spent — makes of time a resource consumed to achieve the outcomes rewarded with money. Time becomes money.

The patient revolution must reject the notion that time is money. That a minute, like a dollar, can be easily exchanged for another minute. That all the time saved is of similar value and that delivering the same service faster is always more efficient. Time is not money. The depths of time are the currency for caring.

I often run late when in clinic. At the reception desk and in the waiting room, time keeps flowing forward, relentless as usual. But in some of my encounters, time flows differently. This happens more commonly when patients and I share stories about the sweet and funny within the mundane and trivial; laugh, cry, and relate to each other's events; build grand theories of the world; discover common fears and common tastes. When we are together, it is as if new laws of physics apply. In these moments, the experience somehow uncouples from the time it should take to have it. Instead of moving forward, time grows denser. In the thick of it, patient and clinician notice each other, and at the right time, the possibilities of care emerge. There is a certain timelessness to care.

More time is not always necessary. Many clinicians will testify about a brief phone call in which a simple clarification was helpful for patients to overcome anxiety or to implement a less frustrating self-care routine. Many will also describe a one-hour visit in which, toward the end, a breakthrough took place that set a favorable course of care for months. Just as brevity can be cruel to patients and clinicians in need of thicker, deeper time, it is also cruel to waste patients' time by being slow and laborious, or by requiring a face-to-face visit when a brief asynchronous text message exchange would do. The point is that time to care should not be invariable, but timeless. Should not be infinite, but relatively unaffected by schedules others set. Whether care takes a minute or an hour, it takes what it needs to take. One visit or 10 years. It should never take more or less than necessary. Because a minute is not a minute is not a minute. Only those at the frontline get to know how much time they need to solve a complex problem of care. Thus, it is central to give clinicians and patients the opportunity to determine — within the inevitable constraints of caring for all those who need care — the duration, and depth, of their encounters.

Patient care organizations must master a trick: they must make time to care. To achieve this, we need to treat the time patients and clinicians spend together as sacred. We must demand substantial justification before anything is allowed to routinely interrupt the encounter, particularly technologies that rattle their can against the bars of their input cells demanding attention and data entry. We must engineer how to save time for care by peeling away all the commotions that distract, automatizing and removing from the foreground subordinate activities that belong silently in the background. There, these activities should not emerge to surprise or distract.

Innovators must be obsessed with removing the industrial frictions of healthcare that interfere with the work patients and clinicians do in partnership. Technology can help solve complex care problems by facilitating and not hindering productive human relationships. Who, for example, knows the data, systems, procedures, standards, and algorithms that are needed to efficiently and reliably raise a child into a decent human being? It would be harebrained and futile to seek consistent results. Raising each child, instead, is an adventure in improvisation and jazz, ingenuity and awe, judgment and humility. I delight in the lovely alchemy that turned my three sons into young men, wonderful in very different ways. As a family, we work through difficulties, bounce back and try again, setbacks made manageable by our ties. The expectation in raising children — or in patient care — cannot be reliability, but resilience. This resilience emerges from the quality of our relationships. Fostering of resilient relationships capable of caring takes time.

Far from responding to the demands of care, rigid time schedules stand as evidence of the fictitious equivalence of minutes. An appointment slot may show a set of minutes, but it cannot allocate the depth of those minutes, the fathoms of time patient and clinician will or should spend together. The stated duration of these visits exaggerates, as some of these minutes will be used to complete required procedures and documentation, most unrelated to any items of the patient agenda. The more proactive patients may play an opening gambit, an effort to give priority to their agenda, but the clinician, pressed for time, will interrupt and take over. Regardless of whether the schedule allots 10, 15, or 20 minutes, the shallowness of these minutes makes clinicians feel deprived of patient care time. If in a unilateral campaign for deep time the clinician was to choose not to interrupt the patient, to lean toward the patient to listen and to understand, and to ignore the demands of documentation and billing, the encounter may still overflow its scheduled duration. The clinic will run late. The satisfaction of caring well will face the disappointment of the next patient who is now sick of waiting, and the anger of the clinic staff who, thanks to the "slow clinician," will now be late for dinner. Realizing timeless care will take more than the initiative of patients or the indiscipline of clinicians.

When I travel talking about patient care, the No. 1 concern clinicians raise is the brevity of the clinical encounter, the busyness of their schedule. When I ask who sets the duration of these encounters, the silence that follows is only broken by some variation of the word "management." There is an equation that determines the encounter duration based on how many patients demand care, how many clinicians are available to care for them, and how many minutes are in a workday. The results are tweaked to hit the income goals of the practice, subordinating the length of the clinical encounter to these goals. This math is misguided. Rather than organize care to optimize a practice's income, the practice should invest its income to optimize its ability to care.

Leaders can start by flipping the accountability flow, making administrators and managers accountable not to payers and investors but to clinicians and patients. They must reinvent and redesign their systems to reverse the flow of resources, to prevent setting brief and shallow encounters as the default just to afford feeding profiteering parasites. Time is not money. The depths of time are the currency for caring. Innovations that add fluidity and forgiveness to the schedule may offer new ways for patients and clinicians to collaborate and reduce clinician multitasking. These innovations could effectively promote time to care well and reflect how much the organization values elegant care. Better care the first time, every time, should reduce the need for return visits and mitigate the unfavorable impact of caring schedules, if any, on timely access to care. Innovators must be obsessed with removing the industrial frictions of healthcare, letting time grow denser, deeper, careful. Letting care happen.

I recognize that it is hard to get both timely access to care and high-quality care. But we must try. Access to poor care may do more harm than good and undermine trust in patient care; inaccessible high-quality care is violently unjust — both demoralize clinicians and patients. Reducing waste, particularly administrative waste, and profit may make additional resources available to manage the tradeoff between access to and quality of care. In improving efficiency, however, we must respect time for care: a minute is not a minute is not a minute. Not all efficiencies can be achieved without hurting care. Rushing — doing a lot in little time — can "deliver care" in little time, a favorable productivity statistic of no value to the patient or the clinician if this care is ineffective. The efficient clinic is elegant, not cheap.

Healthcare efficiency is important, but pursuing efficiencies in the work patients must do is most important. It is the patient's time, energy, and attention that are especially scarce and that we need to kindly respect. We must strive to ensure that accessing and using care causes the least disruption to patient lives. In these lives, a more important and fundamental saga awaits to play out: the pursuit of their hopes and dreams amidst disappointment and misfortune. Our careful care must alleviate this saga from the burden of illness; our kindness must free it from the hindrance of health care. This starts by letting time for care grow denser and deeper.

Timeless care. The clock respectfully waits.

Two boats come down the canal and approach each other. Lines thrown from each one to the other now moor them together.

— Permission to board, says the clinician, eager.
— Permission granted, says the patient, hopeful.

A candle is lit on a small round table, breaking the darkness. A bit of wind, almost no wake in the water.

The clinician breaks the silence. "What is on your mind?"

Two boats swing in unison side by side. A human noticing another. Care.

Time stands still. Time flies.

Careful

My frustration must not show as I review her list of 12 medications, three of them for diabetes. Ms. Olson seemed quite able to control her blood sugar levels with one drug, a sensible diet, and pleasurable activity. I asked why she was taking the two new drugs for diabetes. "My doctor wanted my sugar levels to be close to normal." Some of these medications were causing low blood sugars, which she was not detecting well. They were probably why she was getting confused, not Alzheimer's, as she feared.

Again, I asked why. "He said that my nerves and blood vessels need normal sugars to work well." After 12 years of mild diabetes, at 64, at low risk of heart troubles and free of diabetes complications, I judged the treatment escalation and its unpleasant effects unnecessary. I kept the next why to myself.

Gone are the days in which treatments were "secret formulae," the product of personal (and unpublished) research or expressions of medical art. For most conditions, the range of treatment options is known and available, and any variation in care should respond to differences in what patients need and want. This leaves no good reason why a particular patient should receive different treatments for the same condition from different clinicians, but it happens. The contemporary answer is in the stories clinicians use to justify these treatments to themselves and to their patients. Sometimes, clinicians tell stories about biological mechanisms of cause and effect, brought to the bedside from the basic science bench. They are elegant, beautiful, and compelling stories. "For this patient's blood vessels and nerves to work well, they need to be bathed in blood with normal levels of sugar." Perhaps true, but perhaps not: this story's punchline does not reliably predict whether patients who normalize their sugars with treatment will avoid diabetes complications. For that, we need clinical trials.

Over the last 40 years, clinical trials with more than 40,000 patients with type 2 diabetes have found that lowering sugars to some extent (nowhere near the normal levels Ms. Olson' doctor advocated) helps prevent heart attacks (reducing that risk — in relative terms — by 15 percent, from 20 heart attacks in every 100 untreated patients to 17 in 100 treated ones — in absolute terms that is three fewer heart attacks in 10 years), and avoid the debilitating symptoms of high blood sugars (fatigue, thirst, excessive urination, hunger, and weight loss). This body of work has not been able to convincingly demonstrate any benefit of normalizing sugar levels on the prevention of other diabetes complications. Control sugars tighter, though, and you increase the cost, complexity, and side effects of treatment. These often include weight gain and low blood sugar reactions, reactions that some patients experience as near-death. Given the limited potential benefit and substantial harms and inconveniences, why subject Ms. Olson and others like her to more treatment?

Patient care should be careful, and its actions should be competent and cautious. Its goal, to advance the human situation of each patient, should be pursued with concern and compassion. Careful care requires clinicians to work with each patient to develop a clear understanding of the patient's situation and to diagnose which aspect of the situation requires action. Using the best science to make evident the alternative paths forward, patient and clinician test the treatment options to see how well each one responds to what the situation demands. When the way forward that makes the most sense — intellectual, emotional, and practical sense — emerges, they implement it, securing the necessary resources to make it work safely. If completely successful, care should enable patients to be and do, minimally hindered by illness and treatment.

Using the best science

For most of the 20th century, the credibility of a practice was predicated on the authority and charisma of the teacher and the quality of his stories. Senior doctors taught how to treat diseases based on "my approach" or "the way we have always done it here." The most gifted would wrap these medical memes in beautiful stories of scientific discoveries or compelling biology. These stories convinced students of the intellectual prowess of their teacher and excited them to the wonders of life and the dysfunctions of disease. Stories would stand as argument for why and how to treat. The awestruck student, when challenged, would retell the story and perpetuate the practice. Chains of apprenticeship helped spread practices and stories, turning lore into the care patients received.

As I was coming of age as a clinician, a movement to change patient care was gathering steam. This new approach, called evidence-based medicine, posited that no matter how compelling the biological story, the clinician's confidence in recommending a course of action had to be related in some way to evidence that the intervention could do more good than harm. These innovators proposed guides on how to evaluate the trustworthiness of research studies and methods to use research in the care of patients. This was deliciously subversive of medical authority. It was also empowering and seductive. As a junior doctor, I was hooked. It was like finding the key to the monastery's library of forbidden books and being able to read them all!

Clinicians who practice evidence-based medicine know they can proceed with more confidence when they draw from rigorous studies that produce trustworthy results. Expert observations from personal experience are not sufficiently reliable or precise. Clinicians take care of fewer people than necessary to draw firm conclusions, remember the extraordinary and the recent better than the typical, and are not competent at fairly summarizing that experience. Research methods can substantially overcome these limitations and produce more reliable observations.

Not all science contributes with the same credibility to our understanding of what to do. Studies in six lab mice or in a culture of human cells are fascinating, but their results may not reproduce at human scale. Clinicians and patients should ignore these studies. We should also disregard headline-grabbing human studies, often conducted with faulty methods that unreliably portray strawberries, wine, chocolate, or sex as miracle cures or lethal poisons.

The most reliable evidence about how to proceed in response to a health situation comes from clinical trials. The best trials distribute participants into groups, each one receiving a different treatment, using a sophisticated version of the coin flip. In these randomized trials, if well done, we can attribute any difference in results between the groups at the end of the trial to a difference in the effects of the treatments tested. Trustworthy randomized trials are those that set fair comparisons (by implementing sufficient safeguards against error and bias) and produce consistent and precise results. These results can be applied confidently to a patient situation.

Clinicians should make decisions with more confidence when they draw from a body of trustworthy research. This first principle of evidence-based medicine should prevent clinicians and their most desperate patients from thoughtlessly running after the next breakthrough, or from using an untested cure outside of a research study, even when wrapped in compelling stories of brilliant biology, ancient rituals, or harmony with nature. Even when these appear harmless — mostly water, say — we must recognize that they may cause personal harm when they delay or replace more effective care, and societal harm by diluting the scientific basis of medical care.

By 2007, it became clear that the 17-year-old idea of evidence-based medicine was in trouble. Our research had found that the pharmaceutical industry was becoming the predominant funder of clinical trials and that these trials' results were more likely to favor the sponsors' products. Appraisal of their methods made it clear that these favorable results were not achieved by introducing error or bias. In fact, these trials were rigorously conducted, yielding otherwise trustworthy results. The problem lay in spin, on how the questions were asked. Spin was hard to detect.

Consider a perfectly designed and conducted clinical trial comparing two antidepressants. The new one doesn't cause drowsiness. The old one causes drowsiness and is used routinely at night to help people with depression who also have insomnia. A trial compared the two but prescribed them both in the morning. Inevitably, it found the newer drug safer. Such tricks — the use of not-quite-the-right patients, interventions, comparisons, and outcomes — reduce the usefulness of an otherwise trustworthy answer. The clinicians savvy enough to notice that the trial answered an altogether different question from "Is the new antidepressant better than the old one *when used appropriately?*" won't be fooled. The clinicians who don't notice will be bamboozled — to the detriment of their patients. In order of the size of the problem, a host of problems contribute to reduce our confidence in the research enterprise: spin, incomplete publication of research reports (favoring the prompt publication of reports favorable to the interests of funders), and bias. Together, they undermined the basis of evidence-based medicine.

In 2007, along with Gordon Guyatt, I published a paper entitled "Corruption of the Evidence as Threat and Opportunity for Evidence-Based Medicine." In it, we said:

> If clinicians and those who guide them in their practice are unable to detect these problems and alert the clinical community to their existence, the result will be the dissemination of inaccurate (and usually inflated) estimates of treatment effect. Apparent evidence-based practice will in fact be based on inaccurate information. There are recent revelations of orchestrated campaigns that have combined corruptions in the evidence with efforts to directly impact guidelines and programs. The proliferation of "evidence-based" guidelines and quality improvement programs may further increase the likelihood of the naive user falling prey to the effects of corrupted evidence.

The corruption of the evidence impaired the application of the first principle of evidence-based medicine: the better the research, the more confident the decision-maker.

Patient involvement

Guyatt and his colleagues also proposed that the research evidence is never enough to determine what to do in response to a problematic situation. According to this second principle, evidence alone cannot care. Instead, clinicians must consider patient values, preferences, and context in determining what to do.

What actions to take depend on the patient situation, the options available, and what patients value. For most people, the situation they face is never simply medical. The medical colors other aspects of life — and vice versa. Ms. Olson was doing well with just one medication; the treatment was not interfering with her activities as a school teacher near retirement; and her level of diabetes control seemed able to keep her out of trouble. Did her situation require further action? Should her blood sugars be lowered to normal?

Evidence-based medicine requires that clinicians and patients work together to elucidate the patient's problematic situation and how best to advance it. Clinicians must judiciously use research evidence to develop an understanding with the patient of how the available options could advance the patient situation. Here, they would need to understand what impact the treatments to achieve normal sugar would have on Ms. Olson' well-being, daily routine, work, finances, and risk of serious downstream bad events. Drawing from clinical trials and the experience and expertise of the parties, patient and clinician work together to arrive at a conclusion of how to proceed. This exchange, described as a conversational dance and called shared decision-making, remains — unfortunately — rare.

Shared decision-making is an empathic conversation by which patient and clinician think, talk, and feel through the situation and test evidence-based options against the patient's situation. Shared decision-making helps to avoid the tyranny of evidence — of doing what the study found was best, regardless of who the patient is — and promotes care that fits each person. It is not giving patients what they want, as if they were consumers or as customers of our business. It is not giving patients information or a menu full of choices and leaving them alone to sort out what is best for them. Shared decision-making is a human expression of care.

Facing elevated blood sugar levels, some patients, not greatly bothered by the prospect of more treatment, placing a high value on achieving a small reduction in the risk of heart attacks, and hopeful that eventually this strategy will have other benefits, might choose to normalize these sugar levels. Others, like Ms. Olson, will find no reason to intensify her treatment to achieve those levels. But she did not get a chance to realize that.

Ms. Olson probably assumed that there was a technically correct answer, the right thing to do *for people like her*. An answer that is correct regardless of *who you are* would also need everyone to value the same things to the same degree. This happens rarely. Or perhaps Ms. Olson assumed her clinician knew her well enough to make a recommendation without involving her. This may happen when patient and clinician have enjoyed a long-term relationship. Yet, even then, it would be arrogant for clinicians to confuse a series of 15-minute appointments with a patient with knowing and understanding that person.

Although Ms. Olson is most expert about herself, she recognizes and trusts her clinician's expertise and judgment. Clinicians, however, appear much less ready to consider the experiences, knowledge, and views of the patient in formulating a plan of action. They wish patients would not confuse a series of 15-minute online searches with knowing and understanding medicine. When clinicians attempt to involve patients, they often discourage their engagement inadvertently by using medical jargon. They sometimes offer recommendations without noting other options or discussing the merits. Ms. Olson' care was not shaped by her own views, and now her care — taking three instead of one pill and having many low-blood-sugar reactions that scare her and impair her function — makes little intellectual, emotional, and practical sense to her.

Why did Ms. Olson end up with a treatment that made no sense for her? For an explanation, we may need to explore how medicine forgot the second principle of evidence-based medicine, instead turning to cookbook medicine for recipes for *patients like this* in lieu of care for *this patient*. A cottage industry of specialty societies and disease organizations — such as the American College of Cardiology and the American Diabetes Association — began to produce practice guidelines with testing and treatment recommendations for clinicians. Guidelines and recommendations do not sound too controlling — and they needn't be, particularly when the guidelines differentiate between "right for all" and "right for some but not all." Presumably, clinicians should, and if they understand caring medicine would, individualize their guidance to each person.

A second cottage industry emerged, one that held clinicians accountable to following guidelines. Policymakers selected easy-to-collect markers of guideline adherence of dubious importance — easy to collect electronically but of limited meaning to patients — and used these to judge the quality of care. Their application was mostly context free and the carrots and sticks payers linked to them, such as handing out or withholding money, had the effect of discouraging clinicians from using discretion. Industrial healthcare deployed a degraded version of evidence-based medicine to hold clinicians accountable for complying with what was recommended for *patients like this*, not for figuring out what was best *for this patient*.

Furthermore, technical and professional arrogance, heavy marketing of tests and treatments, incentives to promote procedures and devices, policies that limit the range of options or make clinicians pay when they select a more expensive option, along with time constraints, further inhibit, impair, or sabotage the conversations patients and clinicians must have to figure out how best to advance each patient's situation.

I hit the road and discussed these issues candidly with clinicians. In my presentation entitled "The End of EBM," I presented how industrial interests introduced error, bias, fraud, spin, and selective publication to corrupt the evidence in their favor. Then I noted that, after much work to promote patient involvement in making decisions, this practice remained a unicorn. When patient involvement happened, it was either a labor of love against protocol or a happy accident. The corruption of the evidence and its use, blind and deaf to patient values and context, meant to me that perhaps evidence-based medicine had failed. That it was possibly the end.

I did not want my presentation to play like an arthouse film: Girl and boy meet and fall in love, and just as they are about to kiss for the first time, they walk away. Fade to black. Roll credits. Here, I see hope for a happier ending.

The way forward

We cannot let evidence-based medicine come to its end as collateral damage of the progress of industrial healthcare. We cannot let protocols, algorithms, policies, artificial intelligence, avatars, or who knows what other decision-making monsters pretend evidence alone can care. We cannot let these technologies, incapable of practical wisdom, replace our judgments and displace our partnerships. We must prevent the tyranny of evidence from abolishing our conversations and killing our dances.

Failure to mobilize will further demean our clinicians, drown their empathy, and sabotage their ability to care. Failure to act will enable the ongoing corruption of healthcare's caring mission, placing patients and their care as means to industrial ends, alienating patients or admitting them to a system capable of cruelty. We do not want a healthcare industry. We want, and must fight for, careful patient care.

Careful patient care starts with noticing. This is a key factor in the success of charlatans and faux healers. They listen actively. They see the person. They notice. Patients feel cared for. This is true — even when the care is technically nothing more than an elaborate ritual or when it carries a high likelihood of harm. Thus, after noticing, clinicians must respond by practicing evidence-based medicine.

I find hope in furthering the revolutionary idea of evidence-based medicine, not in discarding it. In fact, evidence-based medicine has been successful at uncovering the corruption of the evidence. To uproot corruption, many campaigns are underway to promote stakeholder participation in formulating questions and conducting research and to fully report all study methods and results. A patient revolution must advocate for these and other initiatives that support and promote the independent funding, conduct, and full publication of the science of fair and pertinent evaluations and comparisons.

Systems, algorithms, and guidelines must draw from the most trustworthy research available to make care effective and safe. Except for safety procedures, these tools should stay outside of the clinical encounter. If they must enter this sacred space, they should stand by, ready to guide and support without interrupting, distracting, or overwhelming the attention of clinicians and patients. Their implementation must be cautious, never incentivized financially, and only after rigorous testing to make sure that they offer a favorable balance of intended and unintended effects.

Evidence-based medicine cannot contribute to careful care without accounting for the unique situations patients face. The human ability to address these problems in conversation must be protected and enhanced. The patient revolution must create the opportunities, eliminate distractions, and give more minutes and fathoms of time for these conversations to proceed elegantly. In these spaces, clinicians can invite, guide, explain, lead the discussion — or follow the patient's leadership. Patients can gather the presence, amidst suffering and uncertainty, to take part. As experts in their own circumstance, they must work with clinicians to uncover the nuances of their situation and discover the best way through it. Shared decision-making researchers are beginning to identify ways to promote these conversations during the clinical encounter, to integrate them into clinic policies and workflows, and to design them properly so that shared decision-making is more regularly present in usual care.

In 2007, I was declaring the end of evidence-based medicine. In 2017, the situation calls for a movement, a revolution for competent and cautious care, pursued with concern and compassion. It will not happen naturally or spontaneously. History has shown us that progress will be demanding, but we must fight for trustworthy evidence, elegant consultations, and shared decision-making dances.

92

We pressed the "Play" button.

The video showed them finding their spots in the office.

The clinician slumped down, logged onto the computer, and turned right to face the patient. His head and the weight of the world rested on the palm of his left hand.

"Good to see you," said the clinician, toneless, tired.

The patient grunted, his hips digging, mining the sofa for a comfortable spot.

Our research camera peered at the patient's face from behind the clinician.

The 92-year-old man was in the office to discuss his diabetes. His high blood sugars were causing fatigue. Diet and activity were of no help. Patient and clinician were participating in our test of a tool designed to assist them with figuring out how to respond to this situation. The tool, a series of issue cards, shows how the available diabetes medicines differ in ways that matter to patients.

"What aspect of your next diabetes medication would you like to discuss first?" The clinician followed the script.

The patient quickly pointed at one of the cards, "Weight change!"

The clinician's head left the palm, "Why?" His body, now upright, pivoted completely to face the patient and away from the camera. "You are 92," he added. "Why do you care about your weight?"

"My wife died six months ago," he said. "That was sad."

The clinician assented, leaning forward.

"My dog died three months ago," the patient continued. "That was a tragedy."

This time, the camera caught a subtle elevation of the right angle of the patient's mouth, a coquettish micro-smile. "I am moving to an assisted living facility for old folks like me," he added.

"Yes ..." whispered the clinician, inviting him to continue.

"Doc ..."

"Yes?"

They both now leaned toward each other, as if in sharing a secret.

"That place is filled with women!"

Patient and clinician laughed, making eye contact. After a decade of knowing each other, they had started to cover new ground.

In the "Weight Change" card, the patient found a medication able to help him lose weight. "That one," he selected.

"Ok," said the clinician amused and curious, "what aspect of that medication would you want to learn about next?"

The next card selected, "Daily Routine," described that this drug required two injections every day.

"Perfect!" said the patient sitting back, beaming.

"What?" The clinician could not contain himself. "Why would you want to take injections at this stage of your life? Why not one of these pills?"

"Doc," he said softly, leaning forward as if sharing another secret. The camera captured the light coming from the mischievous twinkle in his eyes.

"Yes?"

"The nurse comes twice a day to give it to you!"

Belly laughs filled the room and saturated the recording. Their laughter, in sync now, the sound of their complicity erasing their 45-year gap.

After the tape stopped, the clinician wrote the prescription and referred the patient for diabetes education. The patient's medication benefits plan rejected the prescription, but the clinician, doing his part, insisted by preparing and submitting multiple letters and forms until he got it approved. Armed with the new drug, the patient went to see the specialty nurse, but the appointment was scheduled with a diabetes specialist by mistake.

"So, *who* decided to put you on this medication?" the specialist asked incredulous, nonverbally asking for the incompetent idiot's name.

"My doctor and I," said the patient, doing his part. "But it was mostly my idea. You see, my wife died six months ago."

Conversations

In 2016, I gave more than 70 presentations about patient care and the burden of treatment on patients. At the end of these conversations, mostly with clinicians, the first question they almost always asked was, "What about our burden of work? We don't have time to care in the way you describe. What can we do?" I expected this question every time, yet it never failed to take me aback. "Patients," I would say, my smile intended to prepare them for a friendly challenge, "think you are in charge. And you tell me you don't control your schedule. Who is in charge here?" Although I have made this point multiple times, only now, in writing this, have I come to a more complete appreciation of what "not being in charge" means to patients and clinicians.

Care is what patients and clinicians create. You can read about dance, hear the music, and see a chart with the steps, but dancing starts and ends with the dancers' bodies responding to the music and to each other. You can be thrilled by their moves, but catch the dancers' eyes and you will have to accept that only they are dancing. Care is intimate. As it helps the sufferer, care is beautiful. Imagine the despair these clinicians and their patients feel when they realize they have no control over the music, that others determine the choreography.

Why are the dancers of care feeling alienated, unable to shape the when and how of their dances? Why is the opportunity for careful and kind care a welcomed accident? Just as healthcare turned its caring mission on its head and made care the means to achieve corporate ends, it also, to be consistent I guess, flipped the chain of accountability.

"Delivering" care is how the system produces value. Clinicians are accountable for delivering care and producing outcomes, which requires patients to do their part. Patients must work *for* their clinician. Some patients quit or delay appointments to avoid having to report and explain to the clinician-turned-factory boss how it is that they could not complete the work assigned. The clinician may then want to "engage" and "activate" the patient more, threaten the patient with the prospect of poor outcomes, or fire the patient from the practice.

The medical record collects a detailed account of these transactions. Managers use this account to demonstrate to payers that a product of certain quality was delivered. Healthcare bosses speak to politicians and the press about how they produce value to society.

In this system, the flow of information and value streams upward, from the clinical encounter to the corporate office suites and, from there, to the payers and investors. Patients may seem to be at the center of this system, but this is not patient-centered care. Rather, the care that patients and clinicians co-create is the product that the healthcare industry packages and sells and that payers buy. In this factory, as clinicians lose control, they also give up responsibility for the downstream consequences of their actions on patients and society, the hallmark of professionalism. Patients and clinicians are merely instruments of the system with little power to determine the conditions of their work.

In this context, clinicians do not always live up to the expectations of patients who seek competent and compassionate clinicians. Some clinicians may see patient care as an academic exercise, as a business transaction, or as an income opportunity. Incompetent, damaged, or crooked individuals may wear a white coat at times.

Yet, as most patients, I imagine clinicians as professionals who care. Abused out of their professional beneficence, some clinicians join the administration, either to fight the monster from the inside or to escape its effects by spending less time with patients. Others learn to find pride in their ability to follow guidelines strictly and complete requirements. Many realize that this technical practice may fail to care or satisfy, but they feel helpless, powerless, and must comply. "What can we do?" they ask. The abused in the white coat turns abuser, scaring and coaxing patients into "recommended" care that sometimes works and other times makes no sense.

As part of our research, we have amassed a collection of video record-ings of clinical encounters. There are over 3,000 videos, an inevi-tably partial but nonetheless helpful account of this most intimate manifestation of industrial healthcare. Among the unacceptable is the exquisite. With many things to check off the list and document on the record and a waiting room filled with people angered by the wait, the clinician first offered a more intense treatment to meet guidelines of good disease control. Just routine. In agreeing, the patient let a brief, almost imperceptible, hint of hesitation show in her voice or in her eyes. "You don't seem too convinced," the doc-tor astutely and kindly suggested. Silence. Long pause. Totally unaf-fordable silence. The patient interrupts it. "I am studying most days. Working nights. I don't think I can do it." There is no music, but there must be because you see them dancing to its rhythm. The doctor touches her hand. She heard her patient. The patient practices a timid smile, gazes down. They work something out, a treatment the patient can fit into her life, one that makes sense. She gazes up. She stands up. They have a plan. As the patient leaves, she flashes a wide smile to her doctor.

The clinician returns to attend to the computer prompts. She must justify the protocol violation and explain why "quality" was compromised. She must explain why she did not see more patients or why she spent "too much time" with patients. Others will use these justifications to seek reimbursement from payers who, in turn, will act on the incentives and penalties they have in place to ensure this doesn't happen again. The factory keeps going, the machines churning under the pressure to produce. Yet, just before our eyes, two dancers danced against protocol. They cared.

If this whole system were in place to care for patients, would its accountability be set up so that everyone must respond to the corporate boss? What if instead the system placed the patient at the top of the hierarchy? What if the clinician was accountable to the patient? What if all the managers and their bosses, the CEO, the board, and whoever else, were responsible to the patient and so worked every day to advance the patient's situation?

I don't think iterative innovation through the initiatives of entrepreneurs working within the system will achieve this goal. I believe these entrepreneurs may disrupt, but only to position their own companies to profit from a new system, one in which patients and clinicians will continue to be tools in the hands of their bosses and means to other ends like power and fortune. Thus, I think change must come from turning away from this model of industrial healthcare. It will come only from a revolution.

But what would the revolution build? Healthcare based on technological advances is tantalizing. It is possible, I presume, to place our trust in the technical prowess of diagnostic algorithms and autonomous medical robots, and the perfectly programmed empathetic messages from carefully crafted avatars. Their magic could make it possible to begin to experience the kind of love and solidarity that caring conveys when it comes from a fellow human.

Not likely. Care is a fundamentally human act, one that manifests in the dancing art of conversations. This is the art of knowing what to say and when and how to say it. The art of drawing people into a productive conversation and bringing those conversations to a close. This is the art of silences. In conversations, clinicians demonstrate their competence and compassion as patients feel understood, seek understanding and skilled help, and find healing. A revolution of patient care must harness the power of conversations.

A dear friend fell very ill. After months of evaluation, first in Lima and then abroad, it became clear that he had a rare and severe form of blood cancer and he had to get rid of it to survive. His oncologist thought the chances of cure were very remote, but given his circumstances — in his 40s, previously healthy, divorced father of two daughters, small-business owner with almost 50 employees — he offered him a very aggressive treatment program to attempt a cure. After several cycles, the disease did not respond and the treatment caused him great suffering. He could not sleep. He had wounds in his mouth and skin causing him pain. Away from his daughters, but thinking of them, he soldiered on. His oncologist started another more toxic regimen, which weakened him and clouded his consciousness. His lymphoma progressed everywhere, even visibly under his skin. As the oncologist got ready to offer yet another more toxic regimen, my friend's cousin stepped in. The oncologist inadvertently had started to dance alone, and he was addressing a situation that had since shifted.

In a meeting between family and clinicians, the cousin described the patient's situation not as desperately needing a cure, but rather as that of a young man who, as death inexorably approached, desperately needed his family. With every cycle of therapy, he had become less able to feasibly travel back home to be with them. Together they arrived at the realization that the problem was no longer that he had a lethal lymphoma that had to be cured at all costs, but rather that he had a lethal lymphoma and wanted to die in Perú. At the bedside, the patient confirmed his desire to die with his family. This triggered diligent and coordinated work by nurses, social workers, physicians, and his family. A medical plane took him to Lima, arriving 24 hours after that fateful conversation. Moments later, surrounded by family, having kissed his daughters, he died.

Conversations can address what is known about problematic situations. They are versatile tools used to deal with the ambiguity about what will happen. Essential to the adventure of life and a fountain of its surprises and disappointments, ambiguity and uncertainty can also make us anxious and test our endurance and resilience. We may try hard to reduce ambiguity with more tests, for example, but most destinies are simply out of our control or of our knowledge.

My friend's outcome was unexpected and adverse, and nothing known about him presaged it. Once the diagnosis was made, no one could have known how *he* would do — how the disease would respond to the treatment, how he would tolerate its side effects, how long he would be away from his daughters, and how much they would miss each other. As my friend, the patient, was placed on the ambulance that would take him to the plane to Lima, doctors and nurses hugged the family. Then, they hugged each other. Conversations in care fostered these relationships that now were helping patients and healers deal with these unknowns.

The lack of conversations and relationships makes us vulnerable to the vagaries of fortune. Our colleagues have noted, in India and China for example, the increasing risk of violence directed at physicians, sometimes resulting in their death. Take the case of the physician parents of one my colleagues. They were involved in a well-publicized case in India in which a patient suffered a severe, and eventually fatal, allergic reaction to a medicine administered in the emergency room. The patient's family, grieving, mobilized local government officials and the police and had the physicians, who run the facility, arrested without due process. Only a relentless local and international campaign resulted in their release.

Conversations cannot protect patients from the fraudulent, the incompetent, or the negligent. Patients, as anyone rendered vulnerable by circumstance, must be protected from those with the power to cause harm. Yet, for patients in many low-income countries who suffer an adverse consequence of otherwise competent care, there are very few ways to seek justice for what they take to be negligence or wrongdoing. Thus, they take justice into their own hands.

Clinicians are safer in the United States because there is a functional judiciary, although here clinicians are more likely, when they are not able to involve themselves in conversations with their patients, to find themselves as defendants. Feeling at risk, some clinicians order tests and prescribe treatments mainly to prevent a lawsuit and the devastating emotional, professional, and financial consequences that can accompany one. They place their own interests first. Defensive medicine, the term that describes this practice, is offensive to the aspiration and expectation of medicine as careful and kind care.

For patient care to take place, patients and clinicians need conversations and a system that enables them routinely in the hundreds of millions of clinical encounters that take place every day. Encounters ought not to be hurried, but they should not be wastefully long.

Conversation should not replace silence when silence is what is needed. No other agenda should discourage or disrupt caring conversations. The unhurried conversation may be the simplest and most significant act of uprising against industrial healthcare.

Conversations can help patients and clinicians advance the problematic human situations that patients bring to consultations. They can also improve the way patient care services respond to the health needs of communities and how policymakers develop a health care system that is inclusive, affordable, trustworthy, equitable, timely, and accountable to the people. The dance of shared decision-making in the clinical encounter is the dance of deliberative democracy in communities and countries.

It may seem awkward for someone who espouses conversations as central to care, who believes in love and solidarity and in the inherent capacity of humans to notice each other and to care, to call for a revolution. There is, however, no awkwardness, no contradiction. Revolution literally means to turn away from: citizens and patients must lead our societies in turning away from industrial healthcare. We must then turn toward each other — patients and clinicians, healthcare companies and their communities, policymakers and citizens — to build a caring project.

This is not achieved by timid reform or by unleashing forces motivated by competition, greed, and profit, the same ideas and ideals that fuel industrial healthcare. Rather, a patient revolution will be fueled by conversations. In conversations, we will find the new ideas that will advance careful and kind care, rekindle the professional stewardship of patient care, rediscover the old reasons to care for each other, and renew our human commitment to care for everyone.

Cathedrals

For its December 2013 issue, Minnesota Medicine asked me to predict the future of healthcare and describe medicine in 2033. Some thoughts: This is not a helpful exercise and it's impossible to be right. The future could be Star Trek, A Brave New World, Mad Max, or not different at all from today, the latter perhaps the most dystopian. I chose to share sincerely. I thought magically that putting a prediction in writing could better its chances of becoming the future:

> "In 20 years, we will look back at the second decade of this century as the Decade of Decline of the Health Care Industry and the Decade of the Patient Revolution. The health care industry will decline, because in pursuing profits it will fail to meet the needs of all people desiring to maintain and recover their health. People will revolt as they learn the research evidence that should guide their care is tainted by intents other than clarity and accuracy. People will revolt as they see the sick get sicker from too much health care. People will revolt as hospitals and clinics build bigger facilities in response to the rising demand for their services and they realize

*the health care industry does not help people avoid
getting sicker. And people will revolt as this industry
almost renders the healthy person extinct. From birth,
everyone will either be sick or at risk of being sick, and
both groups will be required to consume health care
until or even after their last breath.*

*The patient revolutionaries will demand and achieve
health care for all, delivered parsimoniously and
with respect and competence by professionals who
care. This care will be delivered in a way that fits the
patient's informed preferences and specific situation.
The research informing that care will be sufficiently
independent and rigorous, and studies will be large
enough to answer the questions that matter to patients.*

*Health care will leave the smallest possible footprint
on people's lives. Few people will need it because the
patient revolution will focus on health, on the ability
of people to fulfill their roles and pursue their hopes
and dreams. They will pursue this goal by working to
improve environments, enhance the meaning of work,
strengthen relationships, and reduce poverty, insecurity,
and inequality.*

*The Patient Revolution's success will become evident
and gain momentum when hospitals and clinics become
repurposed as recreation and sports centers, schools,
museums, and areas of social engagement and participation in community life. Then, and for the first time,
they will become cathedrals of health."*

Cathedrals are expressions of what people believed to be true and
important. Families dedicated generations to build them. My own
great-grandfather belonged to the tradition of stonemasons who
built European cathedrals. One gets the sense that to build these
massive structures, communities had to cast concerns for money,

effort, or time in a scale — eons rather than hours — commensurate with their ambitions. Not that there were no constraints: Barcelona's Sagrada Familia cathedral remains under construction, mired by Gaudi's complex design, by civil war that destroyed much of his original drawings and made fighters of its workers, and by recurrent economic crises. The modern construction cranes are as much a part of its profile today as are the towers projecting this breathtaking building to the sky. But those cranes are there, against all odds, finishing the job.

Inside, the light dances between the columns, as Gaudi laughs at our modern efficiencies, our cost-effectiveness, our inattentions, and our hurries. When things are worth doing, when we are building cathedrals or caring for each other, time, more precisely time's duration, is not the measure. Like cathedrals, patient care must be timeless.

My favorite museum in the world exhibits the works of Auguste Rodin. It is a rather quaint place in Paris filled with sculptures, my favorite art medium. My attention is drawn powerfully to the hands in Rodin's work — rough, struggling, with prominent boney landmarks and contracted bulging muscles holding energy and power in them. Those are not the hands in his 1908 masterpiece, *The Cathedral*. Two right hands emerge from the marble on opposite sides. As they come toward each other, they reach upward to create a space between them. In *The Cathedral*, two people come close, their hands calm and soft. The attention is to the space these hands form and contain. That space is free of marble, free of everything really, making room for all else. If the sculptor had not subtracted material from the marble's center, he would not have created that space and the meaning of the piece would have been unintelligible. The fingers made the spires, the hands made the walls, but the space made this *The Cathedral*. Such a cathedral only exists as the hands of two people collaborate to form it, the space lasting for as long as these two people care to form it.

In this book, I have argued that industrial healthcare misses the patient, cares by accident, and is routinely cruel. We need to replace this with a system that notices each person and focuses its know-how and technologies to respond elegantly to her or his situation. This work will depend on bringing patient and clinician together and then removing all friction from their work, quieting all distractions in the hallowed space of the clinical encounter. In this way, sculpting reflects well the work of a patient revolution. It is chipping away at what is not contributing to the care of patients. The main act to bring a patient revolution to fruition may be the fostering of undisturbed encounters in which time can deepen as unhindered hands, noticing each other, come closer to care. We must build timeless cathedrals of careful and kind care.

As in my prediction, a patient revolution cannot be effective without fundamentally changing the ways in which we live in addition to the ways that make a healthcare consumer of everyone and make industrial healthcare the patient's exclusive answer.

One of the most moving pictures I have used in my presentations is that of a castell. A castell is a human construction, a feat of verticality achieved by a pyramid of men, women, and children of all ages, abilities, and constitutions. Many people form the base of the castell: concentric circles tightly connected to keep the towering castle erect and to cushion any falls. A stem rises from this base. A "cathedral" is a castell with eight levels. Five people or *castellers* constitute each of the first five levels; the next two levels are formed by three and two people; the last one by just one person, often a child. While impressive in the heights they can achieve, I use the picture of the base of a castell because it is at the base that a particularly moving image forms: many, in concentric circles, around one.

This picture allows me to speak of the societies we are building. Societies that alienate, exclude the weak and infirm, and make it harder for those most unlucky to realize their capacity, to be and become who they dream, and to do what their spirit demands. Societies that imagine individuals dreaming and thriving, as if success were all self-made and self-accomplished, as if the only difference were that the winner was smarter and worked harder than the loser.

Castells are monuments to a radically different vision, one of solidarity, one in which the difference is that the winner received more help. Castells are the triumph of collective imagination realized. As they grow, castells are pulled down by their mass. When the castell falls, we all absorb the fall and distribute the pain. Care elevates the caregiver and the clinician, but it also weighs and burdens them. A well-built castell, like a well-built society, distributes the benefits and burdens of care, contributes to the capacity of everyone to reach their potential, trusts members to contribute their best, softens the falls, and is made resilient by the tight weaving of relationships.

The work of a patient revolution must transcend disassembling the healthcare industry; it must partner with others to transform the societies in which we live so that they can contribute to our health. Patient care is just one reflection of this capacity for careful and kind care. Along with cathedrals of care in which hands come together, we must also build castells of solidarity in which hands hold each other.

This castell is almost finished. The last one, a precious child, is climbing to its top. Her parents, holding on to their fellow *castellers* at the base, trusting everyone else, await nervously for the music to signal their daughter's arrival to the summit. They are enveloped by a deep sense of care for and about each other; they are surrounded by love. As she climbs, that little girl will not feel lonely. As she stands at the top, she will not think she got there just because of her own effort and courage. For, if she were just to look down, she would see everyone in the village, her whole world, holding her, raising her, helping her touch the moon.

Part Four

Epilogue

Reclaiming patient care as the priority of healthcare organizations and clinicians is our goal. We want elegant care in which clinicians are present and able to notice each patient and appreciate their human situation in high definition. We recognize it will require innovations to achieve careful and kind care. A system of patient care oriented by solidarity and not greed will be necessary to prevent precious resources from leaving the system as profits, artificially creating scarcity.

One of the ways we will know we have arrived is when the polarity of the healthcare world inverts: when policymakers, payers, and managers are held accountable to clinicians and patients. When they see their work as ensuring patient care without disruptions, distractions, or extraneous exertions. When they see patient situations in high definition and work with patients to ensure their care makes sense to them. Today, managers use quality and performance measures to judge clinical care and to document to payers that clinical care is a good value for the money. When the polarity inverts, we will be holding managers and funders accountable for creating and fostering innovative and sustainable systems that allow patient care to happen routinely, while avoiding incidental cruelty. The flow of value will be turned on its head, with every resource dedicated to caring for all.

We must confront the apparent policy choice before us. Some believe in a profit-based competition-fueled system that overserves affluent patients and underserves everyone else. They value this system because they believe it is capable of driving the flourishing of important innovations in care. Others believe that social justice is preferable, guaranteeing universal access to health care as one of the ways in which societies advance their citizens' health as a fundamental right and their capability for their personal flourishing. As with many dichotomies, this may be a false one. A patient revolution must promote new thinking to uncover the ways in which social justice, innovation, and sustainability should not be traded off, but be a joint expectation of any system built on developing value for patients. Nothing else can satisfy our goal of careful and kind care for all.

None of these shifts will take place spontaneously. In fact, my reading of the forces at play is that they continue to lean heavily toward industrial healthcare. So, can citizens and professionals change this situation?

I have chosen to speak of a revolution because reform is not enough. It is time for a *patient* revolution not only because it has patient care as its goal but also because it believes citizens — healthy people, patients who are not too sick to mobilize — must lead the way. Clinicians will join soon, while others will follow later as they free themselves from corporate shackles, relinquish the spoils of industrial healthcare, recover their faith, and start believing in our probable success.

This revolution will not be frictionless, as many have much to lose. I grew up in Perú during the years of terrorism and hyperinflation. I learned then what these two forms of violence do and how they both end up affecting those who are most vulnerable: those who need care the most. The way forward, therefore, must be nonviolent. This path must harness the power of conversations between patients and clinicians, citizens and healthcare systems, and everyone within the political process. From shared decision-making to deliberative democracy, these conversations should unravel industrial healthcare and invent patient care in its stead.

These chapters offer words that we could use during those conversations. As I was writing them, I found myself in situations in which their use in conversation could create an opportunity for reflection and change. So, I used them. They work. I think these words do so because they connect with the values of many of the people with power to change health care. They also work because it is hard to think of care for patients and clinicians when the language is of access, throughput, efficiency, value, reliability, or revenue. Those concepts are useful to run operations and plan the business aspects of these systems, but they must remain subservient to the priority and mission of careful and kind care for all.

It is not easy to access power, to gain a seat at its side, to enter and take part in key conversations, but we must be there. Sometimes the conversations are simply not taking place, but we need them to happen. Effective methods to create and maintain conversations at the clinic, community, and national levels are necessary. To that effect, we have formed The Patient Revolution, a nonprofit organization. The Patient Revolution (patientrevolution.org) develops tools and programs to foster these conversations. It also offers strategies to find a way into the relevant decision-making rooms, including partnering with others who already have a seat at the table and with whom we share the goal of transforming industrial healthcare toward careful and kind care.

Determining whether to join The Patient Revolution, form or join a local group, or act individually is less important than deciding to act, mobilize, lead change, and make a difference. Many established realities look immutable, like the massive buildings that stand as symbols of their power. The only reason they stand is because we all decide their existence is preferable to an alternative, that permanence is preferable to change. Change can be scary and the pilgrimage hard and fraught with ridicule, failure, and unintended consequences. Nevertheless, we can decide that we want a different future and act to achieve that future.

We can all take at least two steps. First, stop accepting healthcare as an industry and your health care as its product. Second, start a conversation. Use the language of patient care, some of which we have explored here. I trust that our cause is just and that we can change the way people think and act with our words.

We can start a movement and surprise ourselves. Like building cathedrals, it may take generations to completely reach our goal. I trust that our work, like those temples, will stand as evidence that we, at this point in our history, cared.

About the author

Victor Montori (Lima, 1970) is a physician and researcher. He works at Mayo Clinic in Minnesota (U.S.) participating in the care of people with diabetes. He graduated from medical school in his hometown of Lima, Perú, and completed postgraduate training at Mayo Clinic in the U.S. and at McMaster University in Canada. Considered "a patient's doctor," Victor received the Karis Award, a patient-nominated recognition for his compassionate care.

A researcher in the science of patient-centered care, Victor and his colleagues have authored over 580 research articles. A full professor of medicine at 39, Montori is one of the most cited clinical researchers in the world.

In 2016, Victor founded The Patient Revolution, a nonprofit organization dedicated to advancing careful and kind patient care for all.

Acknowledgments

Only one name is on the front of this book. That name must take responsibility for *Why We Revolt*, but cannot take credit for it. Credit belongs to a community of loyal and critical friends who understood the book's purpose and helped me realize it. Many of these friends told me stories, recommended readings, or presented arguments that resulted in new phrases with better words. These were invaluable contributions to a book about language. A few clearly understood my intense desire to write this book. Seeing what I wanted to do, they consistently pushed me to complete it. Their love and friendship joined the urgent need for a patient revolution in encouraging me. I hope that by publishing it I have not disappointed my generous tribe.

I am particularly grateful to Maggie Breslin, Jose de los Heros, Anja Fog Heen, Gordon Guyatt, Ian Hargraves, Iona Heath, Brian Kilen, Marleen Kunneman, Sara Segner, Claudia Tabini, and Anjali Thota. They carefully read drafts and offered kind suggestions that almost always improved the book. From them I always heard ¡vamos, vamos! Francine Hedberg generously copyedited the manuscript.

I take responsibility for the cover; the picture on the back cover was taken in the Rodin Museum in Paris, with *The Cathedral* less than 3 feet away. Joy Deborah Robison skillfully designed the book interior. Thank you!

I also thank Norman Bauer, Julia Belluz, Kasey Boehmer, Juan Pablo Brito, Claudia Dobler, Brian Dougan, Catherine Gao, Liz Gaufberg, Janice Genevro, Michael Gionfriddo, Megan Heeney, Jim Hodge, Sreenivas Koka, Manuel Julia, Aaron and Beth Leppin, Mark Linzer, Kasia Lipska, German Malaga, Carl May, Matt Maleska, Mark McConnell, Hector Michelena, Jaime Miranda, Naykky Singh Ospina, Rene Rodriguez Gutierrez, David Rosenman, Henry Schultz, Gary Schwitzer, Nilay Shah, Gaby Spencer Bonilla, Emanuel Trabuco, Rosa Tudela de Montori, Jordi Varela, and Judy Young.

I am also indebted to my work family, the Knowledge and Evaluation Research Unit, and our patient advisors. Your generosity and the zealous discipline that Kirsten Fleming imposed on my schedule created the space and deepened the time to think and write. I hope to have done justice to our work, to the stories we uncovered and shared, and to the depth of your insights. You know how many of this book's ideas and their expression are really yours.

Between 2013 and 2017, I rarely thought or talked about anything but this book. Writing opened me to experiences, stories, insights, and emotions, but not necessarily those from the people closest to me. As a single-issue human, I was insufferably boring. Yet my closest friends and my family did not walk away (at least not fast enough) whenever I talked about "the book." Claudia, my wife, and my boys created a place, our cathedral, in which I found it less difficult to craft sentences about care. Their love, patience, and support carried me through rough patches and blank pages. I could not be more grateful and can only hope this work makes them proud.

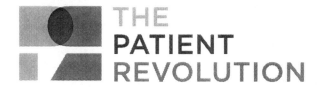

THE
PATIENT
REVOLUTION

patientrevolution.org

Stories can inform, infect, irritate, and ignite a chain reaction that makes the status quo unsustainable.

Stories are the first step in a push for health care that is careful and kind to each patient and community.

Our mission is to arm people to tell their stories and help them tell those stories in consultations and hospital beds, in their communities, and in the rooms where leaders decide policies.

Join us.

At our website (patientrevolution.org), we offer tools to help you tell your stories and change industrial healthcare toward careful and kind care for all.

As you read this book, you may want to share your own stories with me.

Do so.

Send me your stories at:

victor@patientrevolution.org

CPSIA information can be obtained
at www.ICGtesting.com
Printed in the USA
LVOW12s1243241117
557359LV00003B/699/P